Steroids
Lung Di

Steroids in Lung Diseases

Editors

G Uma Sri
MBBS, DNB (Pulmonology)
Consultant Pulmonologist and Sleep Specialist
OMNI Hospitals, Kukatpally, Hyderabad
Assistant Professor
Department of Pulmonology
MediCiti Institute of Medical Sciences
Hyderabad

M Ramakrishna Reddy
MBBS, DTCD, DNB, FCCP (USA)
Sr. Consultant Interventional Pulmonologist
OMNI Hospitals, Kukatpally, Hyderabad
Professor
Department of Pulmonology
MediCiti Institute of Medical Sciences
Director, MANA Hospitals
Kukatpally, Hyderabad

CBSPD

CBS Publishers & Distributors Pvt Ltd

New Delhi • Bengaluru • Chennai • Kochi • Kolkata • Lucknow • Mumbai
Gujarat • Hyderabad • Jharkhand • Nagpur • Patna • Pune • Uttarakhand

Disclaimer

Science and technology are constantly changing fields. New research and experience broaden the scope of information and knowledge. The editors have tried their best in giving information available to them while preparing the material for this book. Although all efforts have been made to ensure optimum accuracy of the material, yet it is quite possible some errors might have been left uncorrected. The publisher, the printer and the editors will not be held responsible for any inadvertent errors or inaccuracies.

Steroids in Lung Diseases

ISBN: 978-93-5466-843-2

First Edition: 2026

Published by Satish Kumar Jain and produced by Varun Jain for

CBS Publishers & Distributors Pvt Ltd

4819/XI Prahlad Street, 24 Ansari Road, Daryaganj, New Delhi 110 002, India
Ph: 011-23266838, 23289259
Website: www.cbspd.com
e-mail: delhi@cbspd.com

Corporate Office: 204 FIE, Industrial Area, Patparganj, Delhi 110 092, India
Ph: 011-49344934 Fax: 011-49344935
e-mail: publishing@cbspd.com
publicity@cbspd.com

Branches

- **Bengaluru:** Seema House 2975, 17th Cross, KR Road, Banasankari 2nd Stage, Bengaluru 560 070, Karnataka, India
  Ph: +91-80-26771678/79 Fax: +91-80-26771680 e-mail: bangalore@cbspd.com
- **Chennai:** 18/8B, Subbarayan Street, Shenoy Nagar, Chennai 600 030, Tamil Nadu, India
  Ph: +91-44-42032115, 45022115 e-mail: chennai@cbspd.com
- **Kochi:** 42/1325, 1326, Power House Road, Opposite KSEB, Kochi 682018, Kerala, India
  Ph: +91-484-4059061–65 Fax: +91-484-4059065 e-mail: kochi@cbspd.com
- **Kolkata:** 147, Hind Ceramics Compound, 1st Floor, Nilgunj Road, Belghoria, Kolkata 700056, West Bengal, India
  Ph: +91-33-25633055/56 e-mail: kolkata@cbspd.com
- **Lucknow:** Basement, Khushnuma Complex, 7 Meerabai Marg (behind Jawahar Bhawan), Lucknow 226001, UP, India
  Ph: +91-522-4000032 e-mail: tiwari.lucknow@cbspd.com
- **Mumbai:** PWD Shed, Gala No. 25/26, Ramchandra Bhatt Marg, Next JJ Hospital Gate No. 2,
  Opp. Union Bank of India, Noorbaug, Mumbai 400009, Maharashtra, India
  Ph: +91-22-66661880/89 e-mail: mumbai@cbspd.com

Representatives

• **Gujarat** • **Hyderabad** • **Jharkhand** • **Nagpur** • **Patna** • **Pune** • **Uttarakhand**

For trade terms please contact customercare@cbspd.com
For general enquiries please contact info@cbspd.com

Printed at: Goyal Offset Works Pvt. Ltd., Kundli, Haryana, India

List of Contributors

Editors List

G Uma Sri MBBS, DNB (Pulmonology)
Consultant Pulmonologist and Sleep Specialist
OMNI Hospitals, Kukatpally, Hyderabad
Assistant Professor
Department of Pulmonology
MediCiti Institute of Medical Sciences
Hyderabad

M Ramakrishna Reddy MBBS, DTCD, DNB, FCCP (USA)
Sr. Consultant Interventional Pulmonologist
OMNI Hospitals, Kukatpally, Hyderabad
Professor
Department of Pulmonology
MediCiti Institute of Medical Sciences
Director, MANA Hospitals
Kukatpaly, Hyderabad

Authors List

Chakrahari Ugandhar Bhattu MD
Pulmonary Medicine
Osmania Hospital
Head and Sr. Consultant
Interventional Pulmonologist
Yashoda Hospitals
Malakpet, Hyderabad

Chetan Vaddepally MD, EDARM, FAPSR
Consultant Interventional and Transplant
Pulmonologist
Yashoda Hospitals
Hyderabad

Deepak Koppaka MD (PGIMER), DM (KIDWAI)
Sr. Consultant Medical Oncologist
Kaizen Hematology Oncology Network
CARE Hospitals
Hyderabad

Dutta Reddy MBBS, MD, DM (Endocrinology)
Consultant Endocrinologist
Yashoda Hospitals
Malakpet
Hyderabad

Kakarla Bhaskar MD
Additional Professor
Department of Pulmonary Medicine
Nizam's Institute of Medical Sciences
Hyderabad

Naveena Nayakanti
Consultant Intensivist
CARE Hospitals, Gachibowli

Naren Bolineni, Satish MS, DNB (BIACHRI)
Consultant Surgical Oncologist
Kaizen Hematology Oncology Network
CARE Hospitals, Hyderabad

Pragna Sagar Rapole MD (JIPMER)
Head and Consultant
Radiational Oncologist
Kaizen Hematology Oncology Network
CARE Hospitals, Hyderabad

Quddus MBBS, DTCD, DNB (Pulmonary Medicine)
Assistant Professor
Department of Pharmacology
MediCiti Institute of Medical Sciences, Hyderabad

R Vinod Kumar MD, DNB, FRCP
Director and Professor
Institute of Thoracic Medicine
Madras Medical College
Chennai

Satish Pawar MS, DNB, (BIACHRI), FMAS, FAIS, MNAMS, Fellowship in GI Oncology (TMH)
Head and Sr. Consultant Surgical Oncologist
Kaizen Hematology Oncology Network
CARE Hospitals, Hyderabad

Sri Charan MD, IDCCM
Consultant Transplant Intensivist
Heart and Lung Transplant ICU
Yashoda Hospitals
Secunderabad

S Lakshmi Kumari MD
Associate Professor
Department of Pulmonology
Guntur Medical College
Guntur, Andhra Pradesh

Sree Sudha TY MBBS, MD (Pharmacology)
Assistant Professor
Department of Pharmacology
All India Institute of Medical Sciences
Deoghar, Jharkhand

Samavedam Srinivas MD, DNB, FRCP, EDIC, FICCM, MBA (Hosp Admin)
Diploma in Healthcare Quality Management
Diploma in Medical Laws and Ethics
Associate Editor, IJCCM
Senior Consultant Intensivist

Foreword

I have always been intrigued by an interesting piece of history. Let us go back for a moment to the first century (AD), when a Roman medical writer, Aulus Cornelius Celsus, described the four cardinal signs of inflammation: Redness (Latin *rubor*), heat (*calor*), swelling (*tumor*), and pain (*dolor*). A fifth consequence of inflammation was described several centuries later (in the 19th century) by German pathologist Rudolf Virchow, is the loss of function of the inflamed area.

History was made in 1948 when the first patient with rheumatoid arthritis was treated with cortisone and soon after other rheumatologic patients received cortisone. Oral and intra-articular administration of cortisone and hydrocortisone began in 1950–51.

What is more, corticosteroids have proved that it can block every single algorithm of any inflammation, and ever since till date, after 75 years, there is no parallel to the razor-sharp actions of steroids. However, like many good things in life, the flip side of steroids and anathema of steroids has been the side effects, proving the doctrine that too much of a good thing is bad after all.

Steroids have a coveted special place in the armamentarium of a pulmonologist in the treatment of lung diseases. Over the years, steroids have been a sine qua non in the prescription for any inflammation-based pathology. The liberty of using steroids for lung diseases extends to other specialties like internal medicine, rheumatology, and intensive care.

Steroids have proved themselves beyond any doubt in the treatment of asthma. It is not an exaggeration to say that in the management of asthma, despite several molecules rolling out of the drug factories, there is no drug yet, to surpass the superiority of steroids. Steroids have made their place secure in every stage and severity of asthma, be it stable asthma or an acute severe asthma and chronic obstructive pulmonary disease (COPD) accounted for 3.3 million deaths a few years ago. In 2019, the number of DALYs for COPD globally was 74.4 million, with an age standardized rate of 926.1 DALYs per 100,000, a 39.8% decrease since 1990. Steroids have been included in the Global Initiative for Chronic Obstructive Lung Disease (GOLD) guidelines in the treatment for COPD, especially during acute exacerbations. Steroids have been shown to cut short the acute phase, reduce hospital stay, reduce hospital cost, increase the duration between exacerbations, and in general improve quality of life.

A worldwide study has estimated that India's death rate from COPD during 2019 was 98 per 100,000 populations, three times the American rate of 33 and the British rate of 31 although the three countries had comparable prevalence rates—3,300 to 3,700 per 100,000 populations. This piece of statistics calls for better management of COPD, including more aggressive use of steroids in acute exacerbations of COPD (AECOPD) either in outpatient or in the hospital setting.

Steroids have played a significant role in the management of different categories of interstitial lung diseases (ILD), hypersensitivity pneumonitis, connective tissue disease-related ILD and sarcoidosis to name a few.

The standard question, however remains if a drug which is good for a disease, can it also cause harm? As the Sanskrit phrase goes *"Athi Sarvatra Varjayath."* Yes, steroids do have side effects, a good clinician knows all the facets of its use such as: When? Where? How much? And how long? The authors in this book deal with this area in a very diligent fashion.

This book on steroids in lung diseases is a need of the hour, and rightly so the authors have put together painstakingly the role of this wonderful drug in different lung diseases. This book should find its rightful place on the prescription table of every pulmonologist, internist and rheumatologist.

R Vijai Kumar MD DTCD FCCP (USA) FAARC (USA)
Senior Pulmonologist and Critical Care Specialist
Director, Hyderabad Chest Center

Preface

We are delighted to introduce this book *Steroids in Lung Diseases*, a comprehensive exploration of the multifaceted role of corticosteroids in managing lung diseases. Corticosteroids have become a mainstay in respiratory medicine due to their potent anti-inflammatory and immunosuppressive properties. While often prescribed in short bursts for acute conditions, these medications can significantly improve lung function and quality of life when used as long-term, inhaled maintenance therapy for chronic diseases like asthma and COPD. However, navigating safe and effective steroid therapy can be a complex task for clinicians, leading to under- or over-dosing with potentially detrimental consequences for patients. This book tackles this very challenge by providing a comprehensive overview of current indications for corticosteroid use in respiratory medicine. It delves into the mechanisms of steroid action, appropriate dosages, treatment durations, and crucial tapering strategies. We hope that this book serves as a valuable resource, refreshing your knowledge and equipping you with the latest treatment guidelines to deliver exceptional care to your patients.

G Uma Sri
M Ramakrishna Reddy

Acknowledgements

- We are grateful to the Indian Chest Society and its esteemed leadership for their unwavering support and encouragement in bringing this book to fruition.
- A special acknowledgement to Professor R Vijai Kumar for recognizing the need for a comprehensive resource on steroids in lung diseases and inspiring us to create this book. His vision provided the impetus for this project.
- We are also deeply grateful to all our teachers, whose guidance and knowledge have shaped our careers.
- We also extend our heartfelt gratitude to the countless patients who rely on long-term steroids for managing chronic lung diseases. Their courage and perseverance serve as a constant source of motivation.
- We acknowledge CBS Publishers & Distributors for their invaluable role in publishing and distributing this book.
- Finally, we express our deepest appreciation to our families and friends for their unwavering belief and support throughout this journey. We are incredibly fortunate to have them in our lives.
- And to our esteemed readers, we sincerely hope you find this book a valuable resource in your pursuit of knowledge and improved patient care.

G Uma Sri
M Ramakrishna Reddy
(On behalf of all the contributors)

Contents

Abbreviations

AEIPF	:	Acute exacerbation of idiopathic pulmonary fibrosis
ATS	:	American Thoracic Society
ERS	:	European Respiratory Society
PFT	:	Pulmonary function test
HRCT	:	High resolution computed tomography
VEGF	:	Vascular endothelial growth factor
BTS	:	British Thoracic Society
ARDS	:	Acute respiratory distress syndrome
FVC	:	Forced vital capacity
DLCO	:	Diffusing lung capacity of carbon monoxide
IIP	:	Idiopathic interstitial pneumonia
GGO	:	Ground glass opacity
DAD	:	Diffuse alveolar damage
HIV	:	Human immunodeficiency virus
RCT	:	Randomised controlled trial
MMF	:	Mycophenolate mofetil
CTD -ILD	:	Connective tissue disease-related interstitial lung disease
HLA	:	Human leukocyte antigen
UIP	:	Usual interstitial pneumonia
NSIP	:	Nonspecific interstitial pneumonia
OP	:	Organizing pneumonia
IFN	:	Interferon
TNF	:	Tumour necrosis factor
IL	:	Interleukins
DLCO	:	Diffusing lung capacity of carbon monoxide
LIP	:	Lymphocytic interstitial pneumonia
TGF	:	Transforming growth factor
BAL	:	Bronchoalveolar lavage
FVC	:	Forced vital capacity
HRCT	:	High-resolution computed tomography
ANCA	:	Anti-nucleic cytoplasmic antibodies
GCs	:	Glucocorticoids
GBM	:	Glomerular basement membrane

GFR : Glomerular filtration rate
FFS : Five-factor score
PJP : *Pneumocystis jirovecii* pneumonia
GN : Glomerular nephritis
MHC : Major histocompatibility complex
PET–CT : Positron emission tomography–computed tomography

Chapter

1

Introduction

G Uma Sri • M Ramakrishna Reddy

The 1950 Nobel Prize in Physiology and Medicine awarded to Hench, Kendall, and Reichstein stands as a testament to the transformative power of scientific discovery.[1] Their ground-breaking work demonstrating the efficacy of steroids in treating rheumatoid arthritis marked a pivotal moment in medicine. This unlocked a new era in managing inflammatory diseases, propelling steroids to the forefront of therapeutic options. Their diverse anti-inflammatory properties have since become a cornerstone of treatment across various medical specialities, impacting the lives of countless patients worldwide. The journey of inhaled corticosteroids (ICS) in respiratory medicine reads like a tale of transformative innovation. Before their advent in the 1960s, the therapeutic landscape for chronic inflammatory airway diseases like asthma was dominated by systemic corticosteroids, carrying the burden of significant side effects. The development of beclomethasone dipropionate, the first commercially available ICS, marked a paradigm shift, offering localized anti-inflammatory action directly within the airways with minimal systemic exposure.[2] This breakthrough paved the way for a wave of advancements in ICS technology, potency, and delivery systems, catering to diverse patient needs and disease severities. Today, ICS stands as the cornerstone of asthma and chronic obstructive pulmonary disease (COPD) management, demonstrably improving lung function, reducing exacerbations, and enhancing quality of life.

Corticosteroids, synthetic mimics of adrenal hormones, have revolutionized the treatment of respiratory disorders due to their potent anti-inflammatory effects. They are available in both systemic and inhaled formulations and find application in conditions like asthma, COPD, COVID-19 pneumonia, severe community-acquired pneumonia (SCAP), acute respiratory distress syndrome (ARDS), septic shock, interstitial lung diseases (ILDs), collagen vascular diseases (CVDs), and eosinophilic pneumonia. Their appeal stems from their effectiveness, affordability, and accessibility, but systemic corticosteroids pose a significant challenge due to common and potentially serious side effects, both immediate and withdrawal-related.

DIVERSE APPLICATIONS

Corticosteroids remain the cornerstone of asthma management, effectively controlling inflammation, reducing exacerbations, and improving quality of life. However, their use in severe cases necessitates careful consideration of potential side effects.[3] In COPD, their role is limited to symptom relief during exacerbations, as long-term use offers no benefit and potential harm.[4] Recent evidence has highlighted the potential benefits of corticosteroids for critically ill COVID-19 patients.[5] Beyond these major conditions, corticosteroids find application in various respiratory situations like SCAP, ARDS, and septic shock, with specific considerations for each. Notably, short-course oral corticosteroids can improve outcomes in non-immunocompromised SCAP patients, while their use in immunocompromised individuals remains controversial.[6] The role of corticosteroids in ARDS is complex and evolving. While some studies suggest potential benefits in specific subgroups, the overall evidence remains inconclusive. Further research is needed to define clear indications and optimal administration strategies. High-dose corticosteroids have been shown to improve survival in patients with septic shock, particularly those with vasopressor-resistant hypotension. However, their impact on long-term outcomes and potential side effects require careful consideration. Corticosteroids are a mainstay of treatment for ILDs and sarcoidosis. They suppress inflammation and slow disease progression, but their role is often combined with other medications and requires close monitoring for adverse effects. In CVDs affecting the lungs, such as systemic lupus erythematosus and connective tissue disorders, corticosteroids can help manage inflammatory manifestations and improve symptoms. However, their use must be balanced against the potential for opportunistic infections and other complications. Corticosteroids are the cornerstone of treatment for eosinophilic pneumonia, effectively reducing inflammation and symptoms. The specific type and duration of therapy depend on the specific subtype of the disease.

DOSAGE, TIMING, AND TAPERING CONSIDERATIONS

The type, dosage, and timing of corticosteroid administration vary significantly depending on the specific lung disease and its severity. For example, short-course, high-dose regimens are used in exacerbations, while long-term, low-dose approaches may be employed for chronic conditions. Tailoring corticosteroid therapy to individual patient needs and potential risk factors are crucial for maximizing efficacy while minimizing side effects. Abrupt discontinuation can lead to withdrawal symptoms, highlighting the importance of gradual tapering strategies based on initial dose, duration of treatment, and underlying disease. Careful monitoring for withdrawal symptoms and side effects is essential throughout the tapering process.

STEROIDS AS A DOUBLE-EDGED SWORD

Steroids, both natural and synthetic, have revolutionized medicine by wielding powerful anti-inflammatory and immunomodulatory effects. However, like any powerful tool, steroids come with a double-edged sword, wielding both remarkable benefits and potentially significant drawbacks. The spectrum of potential adverse effects ranges from immediate reactions like allergic responses to long-term consequences like metabolic derangements and osteoporosis. Notably, their immunosuppressive nature can increase susceptibility to infections, particularly opportunistic pathogens. Additionally, prolonged use can disrupt the hypothalamic-pituitary-adrenal axis, leading to Cushingoid features and adrenal insufficiency upon withdrawal. Furthermore, psychological effects like mood swings, anxiety, and even psychosis necessitate close monitoring, especially in high-dose regimens.[7] It is crucial to carefully weigh these potential adverse effects against the intended therapeutic benefits when considering corticosteroid therapy, ensuring a personalized and risk-minimized approach.

A PRACTICAL GUIDE FOR PULMONOLOGISTS

Recognizing and understanding the discrepancies in existing guidelines for corticosteroid use in respiratory medicine is crucial for healthcare professionals. This allows for informed decision-making based on individual patient circumstances and the latest available evidence. By providing a comprehensive and up-to-date overview, this book serves as a valuable resource for pulmonologists navigating the complex landscape of corticosteroid use in respiratory medicine. By understanding the indications, selecting appropriate regimens, and implementing effective tapering strategies, clinicians can optimize treatment outcomes while minimizing risks for their patients.

By delving into these key aspects, we can gain a deeper understanding of the complex role of corticosteroids in lung diseases and navigate their use with greater confidence and precision.

"Empower yourself to harness the power of corticosteroids safely and effectively. Read this book and revolutionize your approach to steroids in respiratory medicine."

Dr G Uma Sri

Dr M Ramakrishna Reddy

REFERENCES

1. John Glyn. The discovery and early use of cortisone. J R Soc Med 1998;91:513–17.
2. British Thoracic and Tuberculosis Association. Inhaled corticosteroids compared with oral prednisone in patients starting long-term corticosteroid therapy for asthma: a controlled trial by the British Thoracic and Tuberculosis Association. Lancet. 1975;2:469–73.
3. GINA 2023 Guidelines. https://ginasthma.org/2023-gina-main-report.
4. GOLD 2023 Guidelines https://goldcopd.org/2023-gold-report-2.
5. World Health Organization. Corticosteroids for COVID-19: Living guidance Sep 2;2020. https://www.who.int/publications/i/item/WHO-2019-nCoV-Corticosteroids-2020.1
6. The 2023 ERS/ESICM/ESCMID/ALAT guidelines suggest corticosteroid use in severe community-acquired pneumonia (sCAP) patients with shock. This recommendation does not apply to those with viral sCAP etiologies (influenza, SARS, MERS), uncontrolled diabetes, or existing corticosteroid therapy for other reasons. Methylprednisolone (0.5 mg/kg every 12 hours for 5 days) is a recommended option when considering corticosteroids (11).
7. Hodgens A, Sharman T. Corticosteroids. [Updated 2023 May 1]. In: StatPearls [Internet]. Treasure Island (FL): StatPearls Publishing; 2024 Jan-. Available from: https://www.ncbi.nlm.nih.gov/books/NBK554612.

Chapter

2

Pharmacology of Corticosteroids

Sree Sudha TY • Dutta Reddy

INTRODUCTION

Corticosteroids (CSs) represent a class of steroid hormones synthesized and secreted by the adrenal cortex in response to adrenocorticotropic hormone (ACTH) from the pituitary gland, which itself is regulated by hypothalamic corticotropin-releasing hormone (CRH).[1] These hormones play pivotal roles in maintaining homeostasis and regulating crucial endocrine functions. The two primary CSs secreted by the adrenal cortex are cortisol (belonging to the glucocorticoids) and aldosterone (belonging to the mineralocorticoids). Aldosterone primarily regulates electrolyte balance by influencing sodium and water reabsorption, while cortisol exerts its effects by inhibiting the release of inflammatory mediators.

CHEMICAL STRUCTURES

Cortisol, a 21-carbon steroid hormone, possesses a unique cyclopentanoperhydrophenanthrene core comprised of three fused hexane rings and a single pentane ring.[2] This framework features a branched two-carbon side chain at C17 and strategically placed methyl groups at C10 and C13. Subtle chemical modifications to cortisol's core structure yield a diverse spectrum of synthetic cortisol analogues with increased glucocorticoid and/or mineralocorticoid activities.[3] For instance, cortisone arises from a carbonyl substitution for the hydroxyl group at C-11 of cortisol, while prednisolone emerges from the introduction of a double bond between C-1 and C-2. Methylation of prednisolone at C-6 further refines its properties, resulting in methylprednisolone. Fluorination at the 9-alpha position, as seen in dexamethasone, fludrocortisone, and betamethasone (Structure of corticosteroid molecule Fig. 2.1), further expands the therapeutic repertoire.[4]

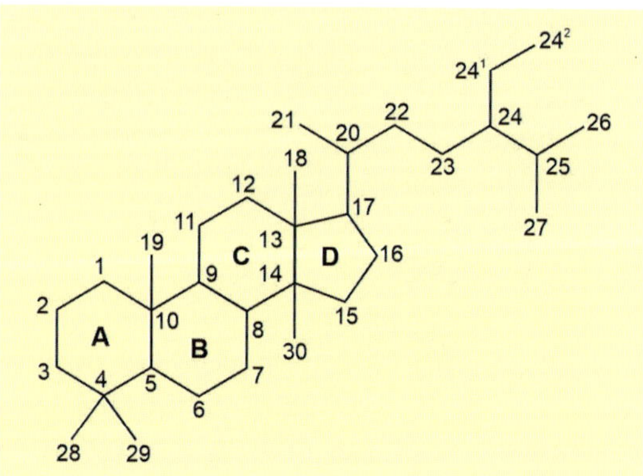

Fig. 2.1: Structure of corticosteroid molecule

Two common clinical glucocorticoids, cortisone, and prednisone, lack inherent glucocorticoid activity due to a ketone group at carbon 11. These prodrugs require metabolic activation in the liver to their active hydroxylated counterparts, hydrocortisone (the clinical equivalent of cortisol) and prednisolone, respectively, to exert their therapeutic effects.

MECHANISMS OF GLUCOCORTICOID ACTION

Glucocorticoids (GCs) exert their anti-inflammatory effects through a complex interplay with cellular components, influencing both transcription and translation of inflammation-related genes. GCs famously bind to glucocorticoid receptor alpha (GRα) in the cytoplasm, forming a complex with chaperone proteins (Fig. 2.2).[5,6] This complex then translocates to the nucleus, where it interacts with DNA in three primary ways to modulate gene expression: directly binding DNA sequences (direct interaction), tethering to other transcription factors, or a combination of both (composite interaction). These diverse DNA binding mechanisms allow GCs to exert diverse transcriptional control.[7,8] While many proinflammatory genes like NF-κB, AP-1, STAT, C/EBP, and NFAT are downregulated through these interactions, GCs also upregulate anti-inflammatory genes, including TLR signaling inhibitors (DUSP1, MAPK1, IRAK3) and NF-κB inhibitors (IκBα, GILZ).[9,10]

Beyond their influence on DNA transcription, GCs can also exert rapid, non-genomic effects through interactions with cellular membranes, cytoplasmic proteins, and mRNA. Recent discoveries revealed that GCs can destabilize cytoplasmic mRNA of proinflammatory genes, reducing their translation into functional proteins. This involves the formation of a GR-GC-chaperone complex that directly binds and triggers the degradation of targeted mRNA. Additionally, GCs induce the expression of the mRNA-degrading enzyme tristetraprolin (TTP), further facilitating the elimination of

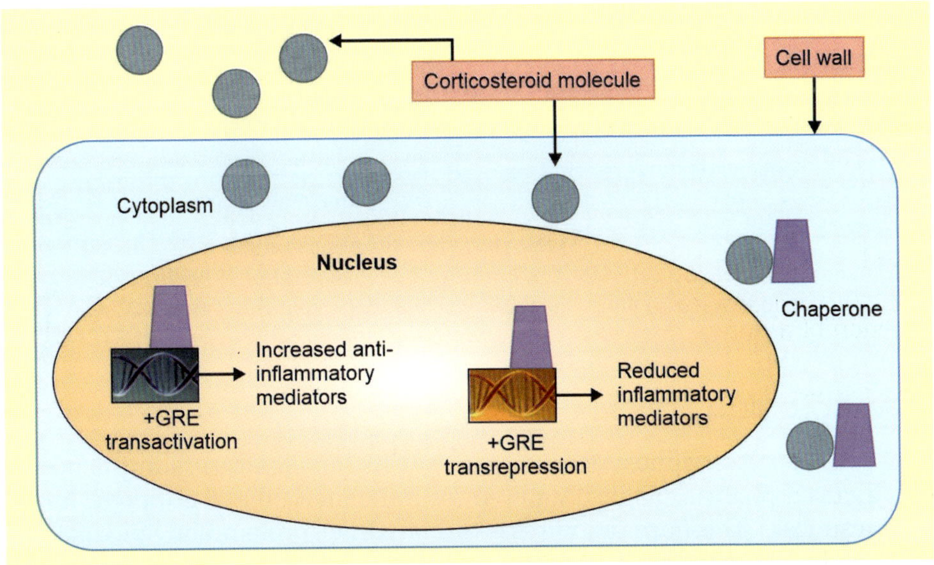

Fig. 2.2: Mechanism of action of corticosteroids (GRE: Glucocorticoid response elements)

proinflammatory mRNA molecules like those for TNF-α, IFN-β, IL-1α/β, IL-6, iNOS, and COX2.[11]

GCs can also exert immediate, non-genomic effects by interacting with the cell membrane. Through intercalation within the lipophilic interior of the membrane, GCs can trigger a reduction in intracellular calcium and ATP levels. This rapid alteration in cellular signalling pathways contributes to the diverse and multifaceted effects of GCs in various biological processes, including inflammation.[12]

CLASSIFICATION

Corticosteroids are categorized based on three key characteristics: potency, mineralocorticoid activity, and hypothalamic-pituitary-adrenal (HPA) axis suppression. Potency compares a drug's anti-inflammatory effect to hydrocortisone and guides dose calculations. Mineralocorticoid activity, measured against hydrocortisone, influences salt and water balance. Modifications aim to enhance anti-inflammatory potency while minimizing mineralocorticoid effects, especially in treating allergic, inflammatory, or immune disorders. Finally, HPA axis suppression categorizes drugs as short, medium, or long-acting based on their duration of HPA axis inhibition (Table 2.1). However, the duration of action is distinct from the duration of effect. Corticosteroids have intracellular effects that persist even after elimination from the body, creating a potential discrepancy between these two measures. Therefore, clinicians must consider all three factors when selecting a corticosteroid: its potency to achieve desired anti-inflammatory effects, mineralocorticoid activity to minimize side effects, and duration of action to define dosing frequency.[13]

Table 2.1: Classification of steroids

Category	*Duration of action*	*Examples*
Systemic corticosteroids	Short-acting (≤12 hours)	Cortisone, Hydrocortisone, Deflazacort
	Intermediate-acting (12–36 hours)	Prednisone, Prednisolone, Methylprednisolone, Triamcinolone
	Long-acting (>36 hours)	Dexamethasone, Betamethasone
Inhaled corticosteroids	Short-acting (4–6 hours)	Fluticasone (FLU), Triamcinolone Acetonide (TAA)
	Medium-acting (14–16 hours)	Budesonide (BUD), Beclomethasone Dipropionate (BDP)
	Long-acting (25–40 hours)	Mometasone Furoate (MF), Fluticasone Propionate (FP), Ciclesonide (CIC)
	Ultra-long-acting (greater than 80 hours)	Fluticasone Furoate (FF)

PHARMACOLOGICAL ACTIONS

Cortisol has effects on almost every organ and metabolic process in the body. It is commonly used pharmacologically to reduce inflammation and suppress unwanted immune responses. This hormone impacts carbohydrate, protein, and lipid metabolism, leading to gluconeogenesis, protein catabolism, and fatty acid mobilization. It also affects bone and calcium metabolism, cardiovascular homeostasis, central nervous system function, and several other endocrine effects.[14] Furthermore, glucocorticoid and mineralocorticoid activity influence cardiovascular function and fluid and electrolyte balance.

Corticosteroids are generally known for their anti-inflammatory properties, but they may also have a beneficial effect on β_2-adrenergic receptors. Studies have found that corticosteroids can increase the functioning of these receptors, as well as reverse the downregulation of them caused by chronic β_2-adrenergic therapies. The mechanism behind this effect is believed to be linked to increased receptor coupling to G proteins, which boosts adenyl cyclase activity and increases receptor synthesis.[15] Effects on immune cells result in changes in the complete blood count and differential count. Glucocorticoid administration causes neutrophilic leucocytosis. The duration of neutrophilia is inversely proportional to the administered dose, with elevated leukocyte counts observed within four hours of starting treatment with moderate-to-high doses of glucocorticoids.

PHARMACOKINETICS

Inhaled corticosteroids (ICS) are a form of synthetic glucocorticoid (GC) with high receptor affinity, making them an effective treatment option for respiratory conditions. These drugs are lipophilic, which allows them to be rapidly absorbed through topical administration and effectively retained in the airways.[16] ICS can be delivered through metered dose inhalers (MDIs) and dry powder inhalers (DPIs), with 10–20% of the dose reaching the lungs and the remainder being swallowed and absorbed from the gut. The therapeutic index of ICS is high due to their small particle size, low oral bioavailability, and rapid metabolism/clearance combined with high plasma protein binding, which results in a short systemic half-life ranging from two to five hours. Though the exact effects and side effects of ICS depend on the drug and patient profile, they are generally dose-dependent.[17] Systemic corticosteroids are commonly used to treat severe asthma, but the potential for adverse side effects means they should be used with caution. Oral administration of corticosteroids can lead to variable plasma concentrations in both asthmatics and healthy individuals, even when given the same dose.[18] The effects of systemic corticosteroids usually take 3–8 hours to take effect, likely due to their intracellular and nuclear effects. Despite this, the duration of action is determined by how long the effects on the hypothalamic-pituitary-adrenal axis persist.

THERAPEUTIC USES

Systemic corticosteroids are utilized for both physiological and pharmacological purposes. Physiologically, they are used to replace glucocorticoids in adrenal insufficiency, while pharmacologically, they are used to suppress inappropriate or undesirable immune system and inflammatory responses. They are used in:

1. Allergic diseases like allergic bronchitis, bronchial asthma, COPD, croup and interstitial lung disease, infectious diseases (AIDS patient with *Pneumocystis carinii* pneumonia, TB meningitis).
2. Indications of steroids in tuberculosis: Tuberculous meningitis, tuberculous pleuritis, tuberculous pericarditis, tuberculous peritonitis, tuberculoma (CNS), adrenocortical deficiency due to tuberculous adrenalitis, massive lymph node enlargement and management of drug hypersensitivity reaction.

ADVERSE DRUG REACTIONS AND SIDE EFFECTS

Systemic corticosteroid therapy wields a double-edged sword: Potent anti-inflammatory effects balanced against a spectrum of adverse reactions and toxicities affecting every organ system and metabolic process.[19] These risks escalate with increasing dose, treatment duration, and specific agent used. From disruption of the hypothalamic-pituitary-adrenal axis, crucial for hormonal balance, to a plethora of other adverse effects, navigating this therapy demands a careful balancing act.

Systemic corticosteroid therapy can be associated with numerous adverse reactions and toxicities, affecting every organ system and metabolic process. These risks increase with the dose, duration of treatment, and the specific agent used.[19] Common side effects include disruption of the normal hypothalamic-pituitary-adrenal axis, as well as a plethora of other adverse reactions.

Side effects due to mineralocorticoids/glucocorticoids: Hypokalemic alkalosis, edema (sodium and water retention), muscle weakness and hypertension.

Side effects due to glucocorticoids

1. **Endocrinal:** Cushing's syndrome (exogenous cushing's), hyperglycemia (diabetes mellitus), insulin resistance, osteoporosis, growth retardation, and HPA axis suppression.
2. **Musculoskeletal:** Myopathy, fragile skin, easy bruising of skin, telangiectasia, hirsutism.
3. **Immune system:** More prone to infections, delayed wound healing, reactivation of latent TB.
4. **GI system:** Peptic ulcer, hemorrhage, perforation, risk of *H. pylori* infection.
5. **Ophthalmic:** Cataract, glaucoma.
6. **CNS:** Behavioral changes, psychosis, convulsions.
7. **CVS:** Hypertension.
8. **Fetal abnormalities:** IUGR, behavior abnormalities, risk of hypertension, gestational DM, cleft palate, and cleft lip.
9. Osteonecrosis (avascular necrosis).

Side effects due to inhalational corticosteroids

Oropharyngeal candidiasis (oral thrush) and hoarseness of voice

A recent study contradicts the assumption that short-term systemic corticosteroid use is safe. A retrospective cohort study of over 1 million people revealed that 21% had received a short-term oral corticosteroid therapy regimen in the preceding year. Unfortunately, starting therapy was associated with a heightened risk of developing sepsis (5.3), venous thromboembolism (3.33), and fracture (1.87) within 30 days of beginning the course.[20]

RELATIVE CONTRAINDICATIONS/PRECAUTIONS

Diabetes mellitus, peptic ulcer, epilepsy, hypertension, osteoporosis, herpes simplex keratitis, psychosis and viral and fungal infection.

TAPERING OF CORTICOSTEROID TREATMENT

Prolonged or high-dose systemic corticosteroid therapy necessitates a tapering regimen to minimize the risk of adrenal insufficiency secondary to hypothalamic-pituitary-adrenal axis suppression.

Drug–Drug Interactions[21]

Corticosteroid therapies can interact with other drugs, and these interactions can be classified into two categories: pharmacodynamic and pharmacokinetic. Pharmacokinetic interactions are often caused by the cytochrome P450 3A4 isoenzymes, as corticosteroids are substrates of this enzyme (Table 2.2). Consequently, any agents that inhibit or induce 3A4 activity can affect the effectiveness of corticosteroids, either increasing or decreasing their activity.[21]

Table 2.2: Drug–drug interactions

Drug	*Interaction*
Cobicistat, ritonavir, estrogen, grapefruit juice, ketoconazole, itraconazole	Increases the concentration of corticosteroid
Carbamazepine, phenobarbital, rifampin	Increases the metabolism of corticosteroid
ACE inhibitors, antidiabetic	Antagonizes the respective effects
Amphotericin B, inhaled β_2 agonists	Increased risk of hypokalemia
NSAIDs, salicylates	Increased risk for gastrointestinal bleeding
Vaccines	Reduced effect of vaccines
Warfarin	Increased or decreased effect of warfarin
Cyclosporine	Increased concentration of cyclosporine

INHALATIONAL CORTICOSTEROIDS

Inhaled corticosteroids (ICS) are synthetic steroid analogs and are halogenated molecules whose potency is increased. In 1972, beclomethasone dipropionate was developed as the first therapeutic aerosol corticosteroid.[22] Today, there are eight such agents available for inhalation. Inhaled corticosteroids (ICS) exert their unique effectiveness and safety profile through a combination of pharmacokinetic and pharmacodynamic properties. Favorable pharmacokinetic features for enhanced efficacy include small particle size, high glucocorticoid receptor affinity, long residence time in the lungs, and lipid conjugation, maximizing local anti-inflammatory action. Conversely, factors promoting safety include on-site activation within the lungs, minimal oropharyngeal deposition, negligible oral bioavailability, high protein binding, and rapid systemic clearance. Oropharyngeal exposure is particularly relevant to local side effects like thrush, voice hoarseness, and cough, while systemic exposure impacts potential long-term side effects like adrenal suppression, reduced growth, bone density issues, and skin thinning. Given these significant differences in the pharmacokinetic and pharmacodynamic profiles of available ICS, careful selection in clinical practice is crucial to optimize efficacy and minimize both local and systemic safety risks.[23]

REFERENCES

1. Van Staa TP, Leufkens HG, Abenhaim L, et al. Use of oral corticosteroids in the United Kingdom. QJM: Monthly Journal of the Association of Physicians. 2000; 93:105–11.
2. Moss GP. Nomenclature of steroids. Pure Appl Chem 1989;61(10):1783–1822.
3. Gupta P, Bhatia V. Corticosteroid physiology and principles of therapy. *Indian J Pediatr* 2008;75(10):1039–44.
4. Bledsoe RK, et al. Crystal structure of the glucocorticoid receptor ligand binding domain reveals a novel mode of receptor dimerization and coactivator recognition. Cell 2002;110(1):93–105.
5. Derendorf H, Nave R, Drollmann A, Cerasoli F, Wurst W. Relevance of pharmacokinetics and pharmacodynamics of inhaled corticosteroids to asthma. *Eur Respir J* 2006;28(5):1042–50.
6. Ye Q, He XO, D'Urzo A. A review on the safety and efficacy of inhaled corticosteroids in the management of asthma. Pulm Ther 2017;3(1):1–18.
7. Scheinman RI, Cogswell PC, Lofquist AK, Baldwin AS (Jr). Role of transcriptional activation of I kappa B alpha in mediation of immunosuppression by glucocorticoids. Science 1995;270:283.
8. Almawi WY, Beyhum HN, Rahme AA, Rieder MJ. Regulation of cytokine and cytokine receptor expression by glucocorticoids. J Leukoc Biol 1996;60:563.
9. Auphan N, DiDonato JA, Rosette C, et al. Immunosuppression by glucocorticoids: inhibition of NF-κB activity through induction of I κB synthesis. Science 1995;270:286.
10. Rhen T, Cidlowski JA. Anti-inflammatory action of glucocorticoids—new mechanisms for old drugs. N Engl J Med 2005; 353:1711.
11. Lu NZ, Cidlowski JA. Glucocorticoid receptor isoforms generate transcription specificity. Trends Cell Biol 2006;16(6):301–7.
12. Kino T, Su YA, Chrousos GP. Human glucocorticoid receptor isoform β: recent understanding of its potential implications in physiology and pathophysiology. Cell Mol Life Sci 2009;66(21):3435–48.
13. Adcock IM, Gilbey T, Gelder CM, Chung KF, Barnes PJ. Glucocorticoid receptor localization in normal and asthmatic lung. Am J Respir Crit Care Med 1996;154(3 Pt 1):771–8.
14. Shaikh S, Verma H, Yadav M, Jauhari M, Bullangowda J, Applications of steroid in clinical practice: a review. ISRN Anesthesiol 2012, vol. 2012, Article ID 985495, 11 pages, 2012. doi:10.5402/2012/985495.
15. Taylor DR, Hancox RJ. Interactions between corticosteroids and β-agonists. Thorax 2000;55:595–602.
16. O'Connor D, et al. Role of pharmacokinetics in establishing bioequivalence for orally inhaled drug products: workshop summary report. J Aerosol Med Pulm Drug Deliv 2011;24(3):119–35.
17. Schacke H, Docke WD, Asadullah K. Mechanisms involved in the side effects of glucocorticoids. Pharmacol Ther 2002;96(1):23–43.
18. Winkler J, Hochhaus G, Derendorf H. How the lung handles drugs: pharmacokinetics and pharmacodynamics of inhaled corticosteroids. Proc Am Thorac Soc 2004;1(4):356–63.
19. Liu D, Ahmet A, Ward L, Krishnamoorthy P, Mandelcorn ED, Leigh R, et al. A practical guide to the monitoring and management of the complications of systemic corticosteroid therapy. Allergy Asthma Clin Immunol 2013;9(1):30–7.
20. Waljee AK, Rogers MA, Lin P, Singal AG, Stein JD, Marks RM, et al. Short-term use of oral corticosteroids and related harms among adults in the United States: population based cohort study. BMJ 2017;357:j1415.
21. National Institute for Health and Care Excellence (2017). List of Drug Interactions: Corticosteroids. Evidence Search.
22. Ye Q, He XO, D'Urzo A. A review on the safety and efficacy of inhaled corticosteroids in the management of asthma. Pulm Ther 2017;3(1):1–18.
23. Raissy HH, Kelly HW, Harkins M, Szefler SJ. Inhaled corticosteroids in lung diseases. Am J Respir Crit Care Med 2013;187(8):798–803.

Chapter 3

Steroids in Asthma

M Ramakrishna Reddy • Quddus • G Uma Sri

INTRODUCTION

Asthma is a chronic inflammatory disorder affecting the airways, characterized by recurrent episodes of wheezing, dyspnea, chest tightness, and cough. These symptoms exhibit variability in both frequency and intensity, along with fluctuations in expiratory airflow limitation. Over time, chronic airway inflammation leads to structural alterations, including bronchial smooth muscle hypertrophy, goblet cell hyperplasia with excessive mucus production, eosinophilic infiltration, and a persistent inflammatory state. Recognizing the diverse clinical presentations, asthma can be categorized into various subtypes, including atopic asthma (triggered by allergies), non-atopic asthma (non-allergic triggers), drug-induced asthma, occupational asthma (triggered by workplace exposures), and exercise-induced asthma.

PATHOGENESIS OF ASTHMA

Asthma can be categorized into two broad phenotypes: TH2-high and TH2-low. While TH2-mediated inflammation remains central to asthma pathogenesis, driven by cytokines like IL-4, IL-5, and IL-13. TH2-low asthma involves alternative pathways, potentially involving non-TH2 cytokines such as IL-17 and TNF-α.

Upon allergen inhalation, antigen-presenting cells (APCs) process and present them to TH2 cells, triggering the release of key TH2 cytokines like IL-4, IL-5, and IL-13. Both IL-4 and IL-13 stimulate B cells to produce IgE antibodies, which then bind to FcεRI receptors on mast cells. Meanwhile, IL-5 instructs bone marrow to increase eosinophil differentiation and proliferation. Subsequent allergen exposure leads to IgE-mediated mast cell activation, resulting in the release of various mediators like leukotrienes, histamine, and additional interleukins.[1] These mediators collectively irritate airway smooth muscle, triggering bronchoconstriction. Repetitive allergen exposure amplifies TH2 lymphocyte activation, leading to chronic inflammation within the bronchioles. This persistent inflammation ultimately drives airway remodelling, a hallmark of chronic asthma.

Beyond the classical TH2 pathway, IL-17 cytokines may play a role in TH2-low asthma. By inducing the release of neutrophil chemoattractants (CXCL1/5/8) and granulocyte-macrophage colony-stimulating factor, IL-17 contributes to neutrophil recruitment into the lungs. Additionally, IL-17A directly enhances airway smooth muscle contraction, migration, and proliferation, further promoting airway hyperresponsiveness (AHR) and remodelling, features crucial to asthma pathophysiology.[2]

TREATMENT OF ASTHMA

The pharmacological armamentarium for asthma encompasses various agents targeting different aspects of the disease. Short-acting β_2-agonists (SABAs) like albuterol act as a first-line rescue therapy to rapidly reverse bronchoconstriction during acute symptoms. Short-acting muscarinic antagonists (SAMAs) offer additional bronchodilation, particularly beneficial for patients unresponsive to SABA alone. For long-term maintenance and prevention, long-acting β_2-agonists (LABAs) like salmeterol provide sustained bronchodilation. Inhaled corticosteroids (ICS) form the cornerstone of controller therapy, reducing airway inflammation and preventing exacerbations.[3] For specific phenotypes, phosphodiesterase inhibitors like theophylline and anti-leukotriene agents like montelukast target additional inflammatory pathways. In severe cases or exacerbations, systemic corticosteroids offer potent anti-inflammatory effects, while immunotherapy with biologics like omalizumab and mepolizumab can address specific IgE-mediated mechanisms for select patients.

MECHANISM OF ACTION OF CORTICOSTEROIDS IN ASTHMA

Corticosteroids exert their anti-inflammatory effects in asthma through diverse mechanisms: Both systemic and inhaled forms inhibit key transcriptional cascades like NF-κB and AP-1, effectively curbing airway inflammation.[4,5] They downregulate phospholipase A_2, leading to diminished synthesis of arachidonic acid and its pro-inflammatory metabolites, including leukotrienes, ultimately promoting bronchodilation and relieving airway obstruction. Corticosteroids dampen immune responses by reducing IgE levels, inhibiting TH2 and B cell proliferation, and suppressing IL-4 and IL-5 production, ultimately minimizing eosinophil recruitment and activation.[6] Additionally, they hamper IL-13 production, thereby alleviating mucus hypersecretion and airway obstruction. Corticosteroids decrease the number and activity of inflammatory cells like eosinophils, activated T cells, and mast cells, contributing to reduced airway hyperresponsiveness. Over time, they prevent airway remodelling by mitigating smooth muscle cell hypertrophy, basement membrane thickening, and goblet cell hyperplasia. This multifaceted approach positions corticosteroids as a cornerstone of asthma therapy, addressing various aspects of the inflammatory cascade.

Corticosteroids increase the expression of β_2 receptors, and this may contribute to complementary clinical effects observed when combined with LABA. A remarkable synergy exists between corticosteroids and long-acting β_2-agonists (LABA) in managing asthma. While corticosteroids exert potent anti-inflammatory effects, they additionally enhance β_2-receptor expression, amplifying the bronchodilator response to LABA. Conversely, LABA not only induces direct bronchodilation but also potentiates the anti-inflammatory actions of corticosteroids by augmenting glucocorticoid receptor activity (Fig. 3.1). This synergistic interaction amplifies their strengths, leading to improved symptom control and reduced exacerbation risk in asthma management.[7]

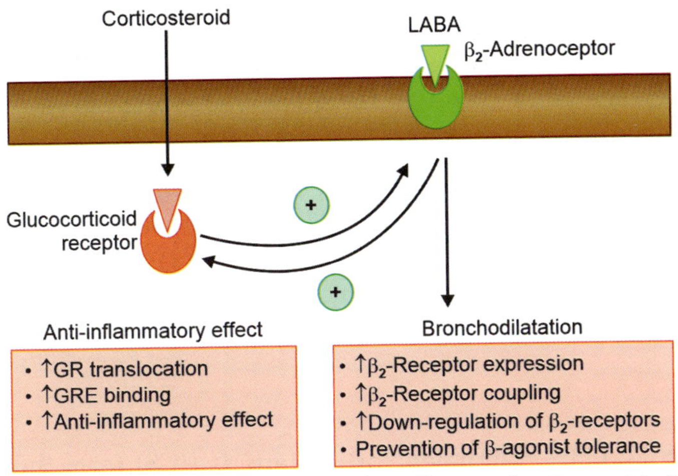

Fig. 3.1: Interaction between corticosteroids and long-acting β_2-agonists (LABA).[7]

INHALATIONAL CORTICOSTEROIDS

The advent of inhaled corticosteroids has transformed the asthma treatment landscape, establishing them as the gold standard for managing this chronic condition across all age groups. Regular ICS therapy demonstrably diminishes symptom frequency, hyperresponsiveness, and exacerbation risk, enhancing quality of life across all age groups and disease severities. They are the first-line therapy for persistent asthma, typically administered twice daily (once daily for mild cases).

Inhaled corticosteroids (ICS) play a pivotal role in asthma management, primarily by curbing the underlying inflammatory processes driving the condition. ICS bind to glucocorticoid receptors in airway cells, suppressing the production of inflammatory mediators like cytokines and chemokines. This action dampens immune cell recruitment and activation, reducing airway swelling, mucus production, and hyperresponsiveness to triggers. Consequently, ICS enhances lung function and alleviates symptoms like wheezing, coughing, and shortness of breath, leading to improved control and reduced exacerbation frequency. While oral and systemic steroids can also provide potent anti-inflammatory effects in severe cases or during exacerbations, their wider-ranging side effects often necessitate stricter use compared to the targeted action of ICS.

ICS is available in low, medium, and high doses tailored to mild, moderate, and severe asthma; low doses provide substantial benefits for most patients. However, uncontrolled asthma or persistent exacerbations despite optimal adherence and low-dose ICS (with or without LABA) may necessitate escalation to medium doses. High-dose ICS, usually combined with LABA, is reserved for very few patients due to the increased risk of local and systemic side effects, necessitating careful consideration of risks and benefits.[8] Inhaled corticosteroids, delivered via nebulizers, metered-dose inhalers, or dry powder inhalers, offer treatment flexibility (Low, medium, high doses of ICS in adults and adolescents are outlined in Table 3.1).

TREATMENT TRACKS FOR ADULTS AND ADOLESCENTS WITH ASTHMA

Treatment of asthma includes a controller, reliever medications, and add-on therapies. Controller medications help control asthma symptoms and reduce future risks.[8,9]

Table 3.1: Low, medium, and high doses of inhaled corticosteroids in adults and adolescents (GINA Guidelines)[8]

Inhaled corticosteroid	*Low dose*	*Medium dose*	*High dose*
Beclomethasone dipropionate (CFC)	200–500	>500–1,000	>1,000
Beclomethasone dipropionate (HFA)	100–200	>200–400	>400
Budesonide (DPI)	200–400	>400–800	>800
Ciclesonide (HFA)	80–160	>160–320	>320
Fluticasone propionate (HFA)	100–250	>250–500	>500
Fluticasone furoate (DPI)	100	NA	200
Mometasone furoate	110–220	>220–440	>440

Traditionally, "controller medications," denoted ICS, are employed to combat airway inflammation, manage symptoms, and reduce risks like exacerbations and lung function decline. In GINA Track 1, controller therapy is delivered with anti-inflammatory relievers (AIRs): low-dose ICS–formoterol is administered as needed (for symptom control, pre-exercise, and during allergen exposure). Reliever medication for asthma can be taken as needed to relieve symptoms quickly. Available to all patients for as-needed symptom relief, particularly during worsening asthma or exacerbations, and for short-term exercise-induced bronchoconstriction (EIB) prevention. Options include anti-inflammatory relievers (ICS–formoterol and ICS–SABA) and SABA alone. However, overuse of SABA (more than three 200-dose canisters/year, which corresponds to more than daily average use) significantly increases exacerbation risk.

Treatment pathways in adults and adolescents are categorized into two main "Tracks" based on the chosen reliever medication. Track 1 employs an as-needed, low-dose inhaled corticosteroid (ICS) combined with formoterol for quick bronchodilation, while Track 2 relies on either a short-acting β-agonist (SABA) or a combination ICS–SABA as the reliever (Fig. 3.2). Within each track, treatment intensity can be adjusted (step-up/down) using the same reliever type. Additionally, switching between tracks is possible to align with individual patient needs and response to therapy. This flexible approach allows for personalized asthma management, optimizing both symptom control and long-term outcomes.[8]

Track 1: The Global Initiative for Asthma (GINA) recommends Track 1 as the preferred approach for managing asthma in adults and adolescents, prioritizing as-needed inhaled corticosteroid (ICS)-formoterol as the reliever medication. This strategy demonstrates superior efficacy compared to short-acting β-agonists (SABA) in preventing severe exacerbations while offering equivalent symptom control. Additionally, Track 1 simplifies treatment by utilizing a single medication throughout various steps, promoting adherence and reducing complexity. In Steps 3–5, maintenance and reliever therapy (MART), also known as single inhaler maintenance and reliever therapy (SMART), employs the same ICS–formoterol inhaler for both daily maintenance and symptom relief.[8]

Track 2: Track 2 serves as an alternative for individuals where Track 1 is not possible or for stable patients with good adherence and no recent exacerbations on their current

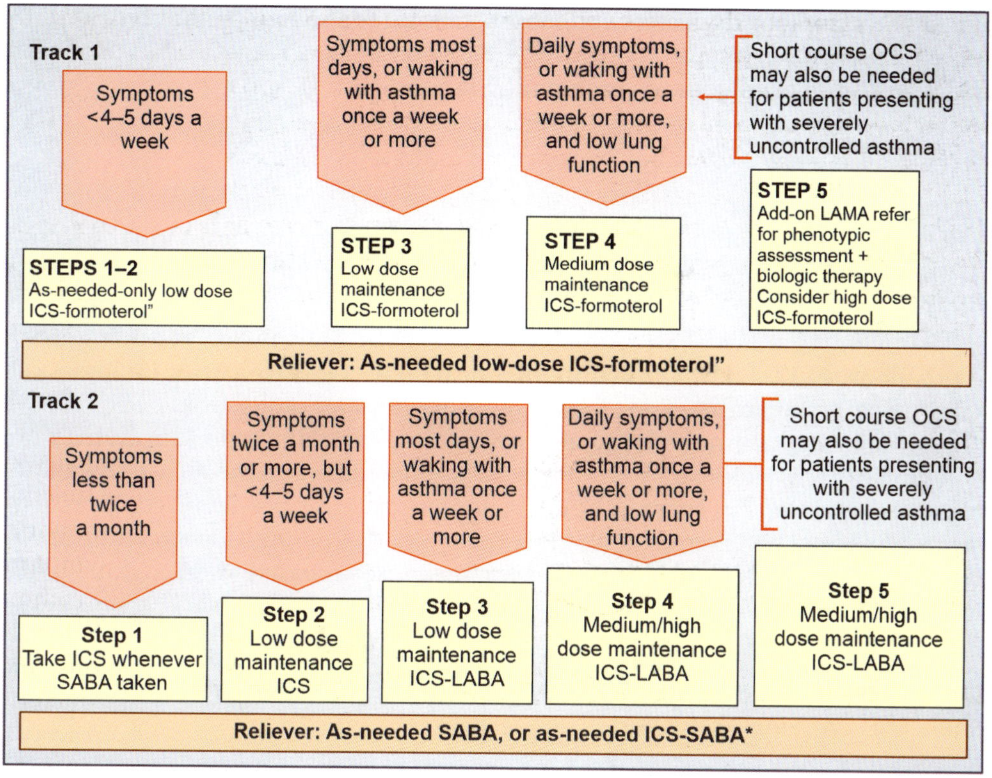

Fig. 3.2: Treatment tracks for adults and adolescents with asthma (Reference from GINA 2023)[8]

regimen. However, SABA-only reliever prescriptions necessitate a rigorous assessment of maintenance therapy adherence due to the increased exacerbation risk associated with non-adherence. Step 1 utilizes as-needed SABA plus low-dose ICS for symptom relief, delivered either through a combination inhaler or sequential administration (SABA then ICS). In Steps 2–5, a SABA or combination of ICS–SABA is used for symptom relief, accompanied by regular daily maintenance therapy with an ICS-containing medication.[8] When different inhalers deliver reliever and maintenance medications, ensuring proper technique for both devices is crucial.

STEPS OF ASTHMA TREATMENT

Steps 1 and 2 (Mild Asthma): The Global Initiative for Asthma (GINA) has revised its recommendations for step-one therapy in mild asthma. Previously, controller medications were standard, but now, a low-dose inhaled corticosteroid (ICS)-formoterol used as needed for symptom relief is preferred (GINA Track 1). This approach avoids unnecessary controller use while ensuring prompt symptom control. Alternative (Track 2) options include adding an ICS to every SABA use (step 1) or daily low-dose ICS with either as-needed SABA or as-needed ICS–SABA combination (step 2).[9,10]

Steps 3 and 4 (Moderate Asthma): In steps three and four of asthma management for adults and adolescents, single-inhaler maintenance and reliever therapy (SMART) employing a low- or medium-dose ICS/formoterol is used for both maintenance and rapid symptom relief. Alternative options for steps three and four therapy include either maintenance of low- or medium-dose ICS/LABA combined with as-needed short-acting β-agonist (SABA) or as-needed combination ICS/SABA.[10]

Step 5 (Severe Asthma): Step five of asthma management addresses severe cases, defined by high-dose ICS plus additional controller medication or frequent oral corticosteroids. Expert evaluation, phenotyping, and add-on therapy are crucial. Biomarkers like eosinophil count, FeNO, and IgE levels guide individual treatment decisions. For instance, omalizumab might be preferred for perennial allergen sensitivity and high IgE, while other biologics target elevated eosinophils. Long-acting muscarinic antagonists (LAMAs) can further improve control, reducing severe exacerbations by 17% when added to medium/high-dose ICS-LABA. Biologics offer an alternative to minimize exposure to high-dose ICS and oral steroids. Six approved options (omalizumab, mepolizumab, reslizumab, benralizumab, dupilumab, and tezepelumab) each demonstrate efficacy with 30–70% reduction in severe exacerbations compared to placebo.[8,10] These GINA updates emphasize a personalized approach to asthma management, leveraging single-inhaler SMART devices for moderate asthma and utilizing targeted biologic therapies for severe cases based on individual patient characteristics.

PARADOXES IN ASTHMA MANAGEMENT CONTRIBUTING TO OVER-RELIANCE ON SABA AND UNDERUSE OF ICS

When asthma symptoms flare, overreliance on SABA inhalers for rapid relief is common, often compromising adherence to crucial ICS maintenance therapy. This is concerning because SABAs lack anti-inflammatory properties, meaning they fail to address the underlying inflammation or prevent future exacerbations. This dependence, regardless of maintenance adherence, puts individuals with varying asthma severity at increased risk of preventable attacks. Even short-term (1–2 weeks) SABA overuse carries consequences, including adverse effects, β-receptor downregulation, reduced bronchoprotection, rebound hyperresponsiveness, diminished bronchodilator response, heightened allergic response, and increased eosinophilic airway inflammation. Furthermore, studies reveal a dose-dependent rise in exacerbation risk and mortality (all-cause, respiratory, and asthma-related) with SABA overuse. The SABINA program investigated SABA use in over one million individuals from five European countries with diverse healthcare systems. They found a concerning one-third of mild, moderate, and even severe asthma patients across Europe overusing SABAs (≥3 canisters/year) demonstrating significant underachievement of recommended treatment standards.[11]

While offering immediate symptom relief, GINA strongly discourages SABA-only treatment for asthma in adults, adolescents, and children aged 6–11. Despite good symptom control, SABA-alone usage significantly increases the risk of asthma-related deaths, urgent healthcare needs, and severe exacerbations requiring urgent care. Compared to SABA alone, both as-needed ICS–formoterol and regular low-dose ICS with as-needed SABA substantially reduce these risks. Notably, the risk of exacerbations and mortality rises with higher SABA use, including in SABA-alone regimens. A long-term study even indicates worse outcomes and lower lung function in patients started on regular SABA compared to daily low-dose ICS.[8]

STEPPING UP OF ASTHMA TREATMENT

Asthma, a variable chronic condition, often requires adjustments in controller therapy over time. Clinicians and patients may collaborate on step-up approaches to achieve optimal control. However, before escalating treatment, confirming asthma diagnosis, excluding alternative causes, and ensuring optimal inhaler technique, adherence, and management of modifiable risk factors (e.g. smoking cessation) are crucial.[12]

Short-term step-up: During periods of heightened asthma activity triggered by viral infections or seasonal allergen exposure, a short-term step-up (1–2 weeks) might be warranted. This typically involves a temporary increase in the maintenance inhaled corticosteroid (ICS) dose.

Sustained step-up: For some patients whose asthma remains uncontrolled despite good adherence and correct technique on low-dose ICS/LABA, a sustained step-up (at least 2–3 months) to medium-dose maintenance therapy may be beneficial. Each step-up serves as a trial, and if no significant improvement occurs within 2–3 months, de-escalation back to the previous level, exploration of alternative treatment options, or referral for specialized care should be considered.[8]

STEPPING DOWN OF ASTHMA TREATMENT

For patients demonstrating sustained symptom control and stable lung function for at least 3 months, consider cautious de-escalation of controller therapy. The approach is individualized, taking into account the patient's current regimen, risk factors, and preferences. Higher risks of post-step-down exacerbations exist for individuals with frequent exacerbations or asthma-related emergency visits within the past year or low baseline lung function (FEV_1). Stepping down ICS doses by 25–50% at 3-month intervals are often feasible and safe for most patients.[13] Before any reduction, equipping the patient with a written asthma action plan and clear instructions for resuming previous treatment if symptoms worsen is crucial.

ASTHMA EXACERBATIONS

Asthma exacerbations present as episodes of worsening symptoms (shortness of breath, cough, wheezing, chest tightness) and declining lung function, significantly deviating from a patient's usual baseline and necessitating treatment adjustments. For patients using combination inhalers containing inhaled corticosteroids (ICS) and either formoterol (LABA) or a short-acting β_2-agonist (SABA) as their reliever medication, there are distinct advantages. These inhalers offer the benefit of simultaneously delivering a low dose of ICS for anti-inflammatory action and a rapid-acting bronchodilator for symptom relief, potentially reducing the risk of progressing to severe exacerbations and the need for oral corticosteroids. Studies suggest that in as-needed ICS–formoterol inhalers, both the ICS and formoterol contribute to this reduction in severe exacerbations compared to relying solely on a SABA reliever. Therefore, patients on combination ICS–formoterol or ICS–SABA regimens may experience quicker symptom relief and a lower risk of severe exacerbations during an episode. However, regardless of the type of reliever, early recognition and prompt intervention remain key to managing exacerbations effectively.

Oral Corticosteroids for Exacerbation Control

For adult asthmatics experiencing an acute exacerbation unresponsive to increased ICS-containing maintenance therapy and reliever use for 2–3 days, or who exhibit rapid deterioration, PEF/FEV_1 <60% of personal best/predicted value, or a history of severe exacerbations, a short-course oral corticosteroid (OCS) regimen is typically employed. The recommended dose of prednisolone for adults is 40–50 mg/day for 5–7 days.[14] For children aged 6–11 years, prednisone 1–2 mg/kg/day (maximum 40 mg/day) for 3–5 days is prescribed.[15] Patients should be informed about potential side effects like sleep disruption, increased appetite, reflux, and mood changes. While tapering of oral corticosteroids (OCS) is generally not recommended in asthma exacerbations, prompt administration within one hour is crucial for efficacy. Notably, severe exacerbations can occur at any asthma stage but are more prevalent in individuals with severe asthma, corticosteroid-dependent disease, and a history of exacerbations (For guideline recommendations for steroids in asthma refer to Table 3.2).

Table 3.2: Guideline recommendations for corticosteroids in severe asthma[16–18]

Guideline (year)	*Drug*	*Dose (mg)*	*Duration*
GINA (2023)	Prednisone	40–50	Up to 5–7 days
ATS (2019)	Prednisone	37.5–50	7 days
BTS (2019)	Prednisone	40–50	Until recovery (minimum 5 days)
Japan (2020)	Prednisone	0.5 mg/kg body weight	Usually, <7 days

REFERENCES

1. Holgate ST. Innate and adaptive immune responses in asthma. Nature Medicine. 2012;18(5):673–83.
2. Holgate ST. The sentinel role of the airway epithelium in asthma pathogenesis. Immunological Reviews. 2011;242(1):205.
3. Fanta CH. Asthma. New England Journal of Medicine. 2009;360(10):1002–14.
4. Janahi IA, Rehman A, Baloch NUA. Corticosteroids and their use in Respiratory Disorders [Internet]. Corticosteroids. InTech; 2018.
5. Durrani SR, Viswanathan RK, Busse WW. What effect does asthma treatment have on airway remodelling? Current perspectives. *Journal of Allergy and Clinical Immunology*. 2011;128(3):439–48.
6. Yamamoto Y, Gaynor RB. Role of the NF-κB pathway in the pathogenesis of human disease states. Current Molecular Medicine. 2001;1(3):287–96.
7. Barnes PJ. Inhaled Corticosteroids. Pharmaceuticals (Basel). 2010 Mar 8;3(3):514–540. doi: 10.3390/ph3030514. PMID: 27713266; PMCID: PMC4033967.
8. 2023 GINA Report, Global Strategy for Asthma Management and Prevention https://ginasthma.org/2023-gina-main-report.
9. O'Byrne PM, Pedersen S, Lamm CJ, et al. Severe exacerbations and decline in lung function in asthma. Am J Respir Crit Care Med 2009;179:19–24.
10. Asthma in Adults. *N Engl J Med* 2023;389:1023–31. DOI: 10.1056/NEJMcp2304871
11. Nwaru BI, Ekström M, Hasvold P, Wiklund F, Telg G, Janson C. Overuse of short-acting β_2-agonists in asthma is associated with increased risk of exacerbation and mortality: a nationwide cohort study of the global SABINA programme. *Eur Respir J*. 2020 Apr 16;55(4):1901872. doi: 10.1183/13993003.01872-2019. PMID: 31949111; PMCID: PMC7160635.
12. Thomas A, Lemanske RF (Jr), Jackson DJ. Approaches to stepping up and stepping down care in asthmatic patients. J Allergy Clin Immunol 2011;128:915–24.

13. DiMango E, Rogers L, Reibman J, et al. Risk factors for asthma exacerbation and treatment failure in adults and adolescents with well-controlled asthma during continuation and step-down therapy. Ann Am Thorac Soc 2018;15:955–61.
14. Reddel HK, Barnes DJ. Pharmacological strategies for self-management of asthma exacerbations. *Eur Respir J* 2006;28:182–99.
15. Richards RN. Side effects of short-term oral corticosteroids. J Cutan Med Surg 2008;12:77–81.
16. Melani AS, Croce S, Cassai L, et al. Systemic Corticosteroids for Treating Respiratory Diseases: Less is Better, but… When and How is it Possible in Real Life? Pulm Ther 9, 329–44 (2023).
17. Nakamura Y, Tamaoki J, Nagase H, on behalf of the Japanese Society of Allergology, et al. Japanese guidelines for adult asthma 2020. Allergol Int. 2020;69(4):519–48. https://doi.org/10.1016/j.alit.2020.08.001. (PMID: 32893125).
18. Ramsahai JM, Hansbro PM and Wark PA, 2019. Mechanisms and management of asthma exacerbations. *American Journal of Respiratory and Critical Care Medicine*, 199(4), pp.423–32.

Chapter

4

Steroids in Chronic Obstructive Pulmonary Disease

M Ramakrishna Reddy • G Uma Sri

INTRODUCTION

Chronic obstructive pulmonary disease (COPD) features chronic airflow obstruction driven by distinct inflammatory pathways compared to asthma. While both involve cytokine upregulation, COPD exhibits a Th1-mediated, neutrophilic inflammation primarily mediated by IL-8 and TNF-α, contrasting the Th2-driven, eosinophilic inflammation with IL-4, IL-5, and IL-13 dominance in asthma. GOLD stages (I–IV) categorize COPD severity based on FEV_1 values, guiding therapy based on airflow limitation (quantified by FEV_1), and clinical symptoms (measured by CAT or mMRC scores). Primary goals in COPD management involve symptom improvement, exercise tolerance enhancement, exacerbation and disease progression prevention, and mortality reduction.

Inhaled corticosteroids (ICS) generally do not offer significant benefits for long-term COPD management due to the distinct inflammatory profile compared to asthma. However, they can be beneficial for COPD patients with an asthma component (ACOS) exhibiting eosinophilic inflammation alongside airflow obstruction. In these cases, ICS works by reducing airway inflammation, potentially leading to symptom improvement and reduced exacerbations. Short-course oral corticosteroids (prednisone or equivalent) are a cornerstone treatment for moderate-to-severe COPD exacerbations, improving symptoms and lung function and reducing hospital stays. It is crucial to remember that steroids are not a first-line therapy for COPD, and their use should be guided by individual patient characteristics, severity of exacerbations, and potential for side effects. The following discussion focuses on the application of corticosteroids within the treatment paradigm for COPD.

INHALATIONAL CORTICOSTEROIDS

ICS Monotherapy

The role of inhaled corticosteroids (ICS) monotherapy in COPD remains controversial, with evidence indicating limited impact on long-term lung function decline and mortality in the general population. While observational studies hint at potential benefits in specific subgroups, like eosinophilic or asthma-COPD overlap phenotypes, randomized controlled trials have yielded mixed results. Notably, the TORCH trial demonstrated higher mortality in patients receiving fluticasone propionate monotherapy compared to placebo or combination therapy.[1] Conversely, the SUMMIT trial showed improved survival in moderate COPD patients with heightened cardiovascular risk treated with fluticasone furoate alone.[2] Though some studies, like one involving fluticasone furoate with or without vilanterol, demonstrated slower FEV_1 decline with ICS monotherapy compared to placebo, these benefits have not been consistently replicated. Importantly, a large Cochrane review confirmed the lack of consistent evidence for ICS monotherapy's ability to slow FEV_1 decline or reduce mortality. However, it did identify potential secondary benefits, including reduced exacerbation rates and improved quality of life measured by the St. George's Respiratory Questionnaire.[3] Overall, the complex picture surrounding ICS monotherapy in COPD necessitates careful patient selection, considering individual risk profiles and potential comorbidities while prioritizing alternative medications like bronchodilators and reserving ICS use for specific scenarios where potential benefits outweigh the risks.

ICS in Combination with LABA

For patients with moderate to very severe COPD experiencing exacerbations, the combined approach of inhaled corticosteroids (ICS) with a long-acting β-agonist (LABA) demonstrates superior efficacy compared to either agent alone. This synergy extends to improvements in lung function, health status, and reduction in exacerbation frequency.

Triple Therapy

Escalating to triple therapy with LABA, LAMA, and ICS offers demonstrably superior benefits compared to other inhaled regimens in COPD patients with frequent exacerbations. Studies have consistently shown improvements in lung function, reduction in exacerbation frequency, and enhanced patient-reported outcomes. The IMPACT trial demonstrated that fluticasone furoate/umeclidinium/vilanterol triple therapy significantly reduced moderate-to-severe exacerbations and improved lung function compared to dual combinations lacking either ICS or LAMA.[4] Similarly, the TRIBUTE trial revealed that BDP/FF/G triple therapy, delivered via a single inhaler, effectively reduced exacerbation rates compared to LABA/LAMA dual therapy without increasing pneumonia risk.[5] The ETHOS trial investigated the efficacy of triple therapy with budesonide in two dosage levels (160 and 320 μg) compared to LABA/LAMA therapy in COPD patients. Interestingly, it revealed a potential mortality benefit associated with the higher budesonide dose compared to the dual bronchodilator regimen.[6] For COPD patients with a prior history of exacerbations, despite continued treatment with long-acting bronchodilators, compelling data from research studies suggest that adding inhaled corticosteroids offers a significant protective effect against further exacerbations.

Factors to Consider when Initiating ICS Treatment to LABA in COPD

In COPD patients with frequent exacerbations, adding inhaled corticosteroids (ICS) to long-acting bronchodilators (LABA) offers significant benefits. This approach is recommended for those with a history of hospitalization, experiencing more than two moderate exacerbations per year, exhibiting blood eosinophil counts exceeding

300 cells/µl, or having a confirmed diagnosis of concomitant asthma (Table 4.1). Conversely, the effectiveness of ICS-containing regimens diminishes or becomes negligible in patients with blood eosinophil levels below 100 cells/µl. Therefore, carefully assessing exacerbation history, eosinophil count, and the presence of asthma is crucial for determining the optimal strategy when considering ICS addition to LABA therapy in COPD management.[7]

Table 4.1: Factors to consider when initiating ICS treatment to LABA in COPD[15]

Strongly favors use	*Consider use*	*Avoid use*
1. History of hospitalization(s) for exacerbations of COPD 2. ≥2 moderate exacerbations of COPD per year 3. Blood eosinophils level >300 cells/µl 4. History of, or concomitant, asthma	1. 1 moderate exacerbation of COPD per year 2. Blood eosinophils level 100–300 cells/µl	1. Repeated pneumonia events 2. Blood eosinophils level <100 cells/µl 3. History of mycobacterial infection

ICS USE AND RISK OF INFECTIONS

Inhaled corticosteroids (ICS) exert anti-inflammatory effects but can also alter immune function, potentially increasing the risk of infections. This impact involves suppressing monocyte chemotaxis, bactericidal activity, interleukin (IL)-1 and TNF-α production, and T cell activation. Consequently, ICS use may be associated with pneumonia. Notably, COPD patients taking ICS exhibit a higher risk of pneumonia, particularly those with advanced age (>65 years), low body mass index (<25 kg/m^2), severe airflow limitation (FEV_1 30–50% predicted), frequent exacerbations, and low blood eosinophil counts.[8] Studies like the IMPACT trial (8% pneumonia with fluticasone furoate/umeclidinium/vilanterol vs. 5% with umeclidinium/vilanterol) highlight this concern. However, trials like TRIBUTE showed no increase in pneumonia risk with BDP/FF/G compared to IND/GLY (both at 4%). Repeated pneumonia episodes warrant ICS discontinuation consideration.

Observational studies in regions with high tuberculosis (TB) prevalence, like South Korea and Taiwan, suggest an increased risk of active TB infection in COPD patients receiving ICS.[9] Long-term ICS use can elevate the risk of URTIs caused by viruses like rhinovirus, respiratory syncytial virus, and coronavirus.[10]

ICS WITHDRAWAL

ICS withdrawal in COPD presents a complex picture. While studies consistently demonstrate a decline in lung function (FEV_1) and increased airway inflammation after ICS cessation, the impact on exacerbation frequency (ECOPD) varies significantly. This discrepancy likely stems from differences in patient populations, particularly blood eosinophil levels and exacerbation history, as well as the use of concurrent bronchodilators. For instance, the ISOLDE trial observed an increased ECOPD rate following acute ICS withdrawal compared to ICS-naive patients, while O'Brien et al reported a non-significant rise in exacerbations alongside a 100 ml FEV_1 decline.[11,12]

These findings underscore the need for careful patient selection and personalized decision-making when considering ICS withdrawal in COPD, accounting for individual risk factors and the potential benefits of alternative treatment strategies.

BLOOD EOSINOPHILS TO GUIDE ICS USE IN COPD

Eosinophil levels play a complex role in COPD management. While sputum eosinophil counts may increase during exacerbations, their presence, along with elevated blood eosinophil levels, can predict a positive response to ICS therapy in preventing future exacerbations. Interestingly, blood eosinophil count at exacerbation onset can even identify patients at higher risk of adverse outcomes, including hospital readmission, poor response to ICS, and even mortality. Trials like IMPACT and TRIBUTE demonstrated significantly greater benefits of triple therapy (LABA/LAMA + ICS) in patients with blood eosinophil counts exceeding 150–200 cells/µl. Conversely, studies like WISDOM suggest increased exacerbation frequency after ICS withdrawal in patients with high eosinophil counts. Notably, individuals with very low counts (<100 cells/µl) seem to exhibit minimal response to ICS for exacerbation prevention, while those with counts exceeding 300 cells/µl may experience significant benefits in terms of reduced exacerbation risk. This complex interplay between eosinophil levels and ICS response underscores the importance of personalized treatment decisions in COPD management.[13]

The CORTICO-COP trial explored whether a biomarker-guided algorithm using daily blood eosinophil counts during hospitalization could reduce systemic corticosteroid exposure in COPD exacerbations. Patients were randomized to either (1) daily eosinophil-guided treatment (37.5 mg prednisolone for counts ≥300 cells/µl, withheld otherwise) or (2) standard 4-day prednisolone (37.5 mg daily). Although an initial 80 mg intravenous dose was given to all, the biomarker-guided approach proved non-inferior to standard care while achieving a significant reduction in median corticosteroid duration (5 vs. 2 days). This study, overcoming fluctuating eosinophil levels, represents the first comparison of an eosinophil-driven strategy to standard 5-day therapy.[14]

INITIAL MANAGEMENT OF STABLE COPD PATIENTS

The 2023 Global Initiative for Chronic Obstructive Pulmonary Disease (GOLD) guidelines introduce a refined ABCD combined assessment tool, emphasizing the clinical importance of exacerbations (Fig. 4.1). While the A and B categories remain unchanged, the C and D groups are merged into a single "E" group, reflecting the critical role of exacerbation history in treatment decisions.[15]

Treatment recommendations for **Group A:** All patients should be offered either short-acting or long-acting bronchodilators for symptom management. For **Group B:** Initial treatment should escalate to a long-acting β-agonist (LABA) plus long-acting muscarinic antagonist (LAMA) combination due to its superior efficacy compared to monotherapy. **Group E:** For patients with a history of exacerbations or other high-risk factors (merged C and D), LABA/LAMA remains the first-line option. However, in individuals with elevated blood eosinophil counts (>300/µl), initiating triple therapy with LABA/LAMA plus inhaled corticosteroids (ICS) should be considered, reflecting the potential benefit of ICS in this specific subgroup.

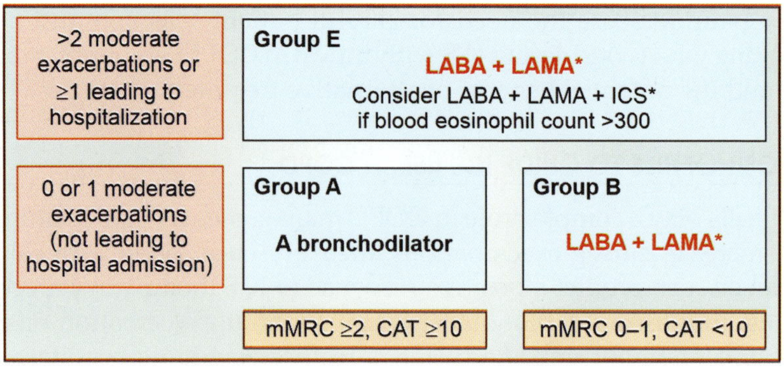

Fig. 4.1: ABCD combined assessment tool[15]

Follow-up Pharmacological Management

For stable COPD patients persistently experiencing exacerbations on bronchodilator monotherapy, escalation to a LABA-LAMA combination is advised. In those encountering exacerbations and elevated blood eosinophil counts (>300/μl) despite monotherapy, triple therapy with LABA-LAMA-ICS may be beneficial. Single-inhaler options should be prioritized for convenience. For patients on LABA-LAMA-ICS who continue to experience exacerbations, adding roflumilast if FEV_1 is less than 50% predicted or azithromycin for ex-smokers can be considered. ICS withdrawal is a potential option if pneumonia or significant side effects arise. This stepwise approach, outlined in Fig. 4.2, optimizes pharmacological management while minimizing unnecessary complexity and potential adverse effects.[15]

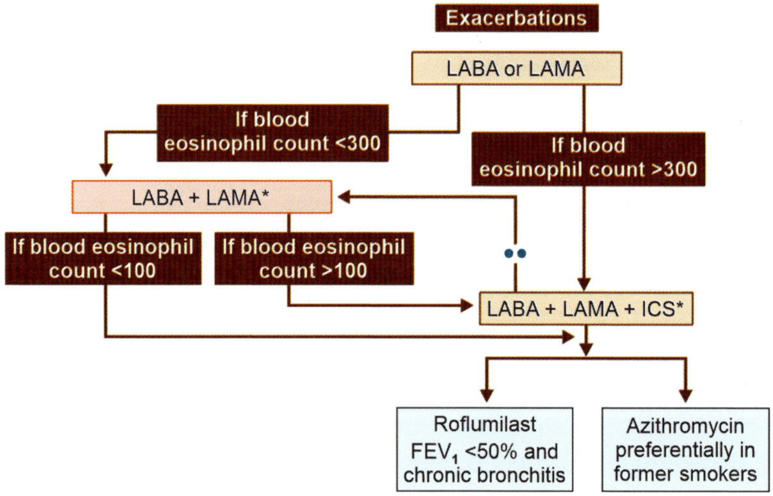

Fig. 4.2: Follow-up pharmacological management[15]

SYSTEMIC CORTICOSTEROIDS

International guidelines strongly recommend systemic corticosteroids as a cornerstone of managing acute COPD exacerbations (ECOPD) (Table 4.2). These medications prove highly effective, offering a range of benefits: shortening recovery time, improving lung function (FEV_1), enhancing oxygenation, reducing treatment failure and relapse risk, alleviating symptoms, and shortening hospital stays. A standard dose of 40 mg prednisone equivalent daily for 5 days is optimal, with oral administration demonstrating equal efficacy to intravenous delivery. The ERS/ATS Task Force conditionally recommends a short course (≤14 days) of oral corticosteroids for outpatients with COPD exacerbations to improve lung function and potentially reduce hospitalizations. While uncertainty remains regarding its impact on treatment failure, mortality, and adverse effects due to limited data, the potential benefits likely outweigh the downsides. Further strong evidence is needed to solidify this recommendation.

Table 4.2: Current guideline recommendations for corticosteroids in COPD[18]

Guidelines	*Year*	*Corticosteroid*	*Daily dose (mg)*	*Duration (days)*
GOLD COPD[19]	2023	Prednisolone	40	5
NICE[20]	2019	Prednisone	30	5
Japan[21]	2019	Prednisolone	30	7–10
ATS/ERS[22]	2017	Prednisolone	30	10–14
Can Thor Soc[23]	2010	Prednisone or equivalent	30	5

While evidence overwhelmingly supports the use of short-course systemic corticosteroids for acute exacerbations of COPD (AECOPD), a note of caution emerges regarding their extended administration. A study demonstrates a worrisome association between longer oral steroid courses and increased risks of pneumonia and all-cause mortality in AECOPD patients.[16] Therefore, adhering to recommended durations, typically 5 days with a 40 mg prednisone equivalent daily dose, remains crucial. In selected acute exacerbations of COPD (AECOPD) patients, nebulized budesonide monotherapy emerges as a compelling alternative to systemic corticosteroids. A study demonstrated its efficacy, revealing comparable benefits to intravenous methylprednisolone in AECOPD management.[17]

REFERENCES

1. Calverley PM, Anderson JA, Celli B, Ferguson GT, Jenkins C, Jones PW, Yates JC and Vestbo J. Salmeterol and fluticasone propionate and survival in chronic obstructive pulmonary disease. *New England Journal of Medicine*, 2007;356(8):775–89.
2. Vestbo J, Anderson JA, Brook RD, Calverley PM, Celli BR, Crim C, Martinez F, Yates J and Newby DE. Fluticasone furoate and vilanterol and survival in chronic obstructive pulmonary disease with heightened cardiovascular risk (SUMMIT): a double-blind randomised controlled trial. *The Lancet*, 2016;387(10030):1817–26.
3. Yang IA, Clarke MS, Sim EH and Fong KM. Inhaled corticosteroids for stable chronic obstructive pulmonary disease. *Cochrane Database of Systematic Reviews*, 2012;(7).
4. Bourdin A, Criner G, Devouassoux G, Dransfield M, Halpin DM, Han M, Jones CE, Kalhan R, Lange P, Lettis S and Lipson, D., 2020. Informing the PAthway of COPD Treatment Single-Inhaler Triple Therapy (Fluticasone Furoate/Umeclidinium/Vilanterol) Versus Fluticasone Furoate/Vilanterol and Umeclidinium/Vilanterol in Patients With COPD: Analysis of Western Europe and North America Regions. *Chronic Obstructive Pulmonary Diseases: Journal of the COPD Foundation.*
5. Papi A, Vestbo J, Fabbri L, Corradi M, Prunier H, Cohuet G, Guasconi A, Montagna I, Vezzoli S, Petruzzelli S and Scuri M. Extrafine inhaled triple therapy versus dual bronchodilator therapy in

chronic obstructive pulmonary disease (TRIBUTE): a double-blind, parallel-group, randomised controlled trial. *The Lancet*, 2018;391(10125):1076–84.

6. Rabe KF, Martinez FJ, Ferguson GT, Wang C, Singh D, Wedzicha JA, Trivedi R, St Rose E, Ballal S, McLaren J and Darken P. Triple inhaled therapy at two glucocorticoid doses in moderate-to-very-severe COPD. *New England Journal of Medicine*, 2020;383(1):35–48.
7. Calverley PM, Anderson JA, Brook RD, Crim C, Gallot, N, Kilbride S, Martinez FJ, Yates J, Newby DE, Vestbo J and Wise R. Fluticasone furoate, vilanterol, and lung function decline in patients with moderate chronic obstructive pulmonary disease and heightened cardiovascular risk. *American Journal of Respiratory and Critical Care Medicine*, 2018;197(1):47–55.
8. Crim C, Calverley PMA, Anderson JA, Celli B, Ferguson GT, Jenkins C, Jones PW, Willits LR, Yates JC and Vestbo J. Pneumonia risk in COPD patients receiving inhaled corticosteroids alone or in combination: TORCH study results. *European Respiratory Journa*l, 2009;34(3):641–647.
9. Lee CH, Kim K, Hyun MK, Jang EJ, Lee NR and Yim JJ. Use of inhaled corticosteroids and the risk of tuberculosis. *Thorax*, 2013;68(12):1105–13.
10. Yang M, Chen H, Zhang Y, Du Y, Xu Y, Jiang P and Xu Z. Long-term use of inhaled corticosteroids and risk of upper respiratory tract infection in chronic obstructive pulmonary disease: a meta-analysis. *Inhalation Toxicology*, 2017;29(5):219–26.
11. Jarad NA, Wedzicha JA, Burge PS, et al. An observational study of inhaled corticosteroid withdrawal in stable chronic obstructive pulmonary disease. ISOLDE Study Group. Respir Med 1999;93:161–166.
12. O'Brien A, Russo-Magno P, Karki A, et al. Effects of withdrawal of inhaled steroids in men with severe irreversible airflow obstruction. Am J Respir Crit Care Med 2001;164:365–71.
13. Yun JH, Lamb A, Chase R, et al. Blood eosinophil counts thresholds and exacerbations in patients with chronic obstructive pulmonary disease. J Allergy Clin Immunol 2018;141:2037–47.
14. Sivapalan P, Lapperre TS, Janner J, Laub RR, Moberg M, Bech CS, Eklöf J, Holm FS, Armbruster K, Sivapalan P, Mosbech C, Ali AKM, Seersholm N, Wilcke JT, Brøndum E, Sonne TP, Rønholt F, Andreassen HF, Ulrik CS, Vestbo J, Jensen JS. Eosinophil-guided corticosteroid therapy in patients admitted to hospital with COPD exacerbation (CORTICO-COP): a multicentre, randomised, controlled, open-label, non-inferiority trial. Lancet Respir Med. 2019 Aug;7(8):699–709. doi: 10.1016/S2213-2600(19)30176-6. Epub 2019 May 20. PMID: 31122894.
15. Global Initiative for Chronic Obstructive Lung Disease 2023 Report: GOLD Executive Summary. *Eur Respir J* 2023 Apr 1;61(4):2300239. doi: 10.1183/13993003.00239–2023.
16. Sivapalan P, Ingebrigtsen TS, Rasmussen DB, et al. COPD exacerbations: the impact of long versus short courses of oral corticosteroids on mortality and pneumonia: nationwide data on 67,000 patients with COPD followed for 12 months. BMJ Open Respir Res 2019;6(1):e000407.
17. Gunen H, Hacievliyagil SS, Yetkin O, Gulbas G, Mutlu LC, In E. The role of nebulised budesonide in the treatment of exacerbations of COPD. *Eur Respir J* 2007;29(4):660–7.
18. Melani AS, Croce S, Cassai L. et al. Systemic Corticosteroids for Treating Respiratory Diseases: Less is Better, but… When and How is it Possible in Real Life? Pulm Ther 2023;9:329–344. https://doi.org/10.1007/s41030-023-00227-x.
19. Global Initiative for Chronic Obstructive Lung Disease. Global strategy for the diagnosis, management, and prevention of chronic obstructive lung disease. Updated 2023.
20. NICE. Chronic obstructive pulmonary disease in over 16s: diagnosis and management. Evidence reviews for the length of corticosteroid use during exacerbations NICE guideline NG115 2019. https:// www.nice.org.uk/guidance/ng115/evidence/jlength-of-corticosteroid-use-during-exacerbationspdf-237699674965. Accessed 12 Jan 2023.
21. Wedzicha JA, Miravitlles M, Hurst JR, et al. Management of COPD exacerbations: an ERS/ATS guideline. *Eur Respir J* 2017;49:1600791.
22. Japanese Respiratory Society. Guidelines for the Diagnosis and Treatment of COPD. 3rd edition. 2010. http://www.jrs.or.jp/uploads/uploads/files/ photos/765.pdf 61. Accessed 12 Jan 2023.
23. Canadian Respiratory Guidelines. COPD action plan. COPDActionPlanUpdate_2019_Editable_Eng_v2.pdf. Accessed 12 Jan 2023.

Chapter 5

Steroids in Interstitial Lung Diseases

Kakarla Bhaskar • S Lakshmi Kumari

INTRODUCTION

Interstitial lung diseases (ILDs) encompass a diverse group of disorders characterized by inflammatory/immune and fibrotic involvement of the lung interstitium. While presenting with similar clinical, radiological, and pathological features, ILDs affect various lung compartments beyond the interstitium, including bronchioles, alveoli, pleura, and pulmonary vasculature, depending on the specific etiology.

CLASSIFICATION

The 2001 American Thoracic Society (ATS) statement categorized diffuse parenchymal lung disease (DPLD) into several groups based on etiology:[1]

- **Disorders of known causes:** Connective tissue disease-associated ILD (CTD-ILD), drug-induced ILD, and environmental exposure-related ILD.
- **Disorders of unknown causes:** Idiopathic interstitial pneumonias (IIPs), granulomatous diseases like sarcoidosis, lymphangioleiomyomatosis (LAM), Langerhans cell histiocytosis (LCH), and eosinophilic pneumonia.

The IIP classification: The original IIP classification included IPF and non-IPF entities.

Idiopathic pulmonary fibrosis (IPF): The most common IIP, characterized by progressive fibrosis.

Non-IPF entities

- *Nonspecific interstitial pneumonia (NSIP):* Variable inflammation and fibrosis.
- *Cryptogenic organizing pneumonia (COP):* Characterized by intra-alveolar plugs of inflammatory debris.
- *Lymphocytic interstitial pneumonia (LIP):* Prominent lymphocytic infiltration.
- *Acute interstitial pneumonia (AIP):* Rapidly progressive inflammation with minimal fibrosis.
- *Respiratory bronchiolitis interstitial lung disease (RB-ILD):* Inflammation centered around bronchioles.
- *Desquamative interstitial pneumonia (DIP):* Desquamation of alveolar epithelial cells.

The 2013 ATS update revised the IIP classification, incorporating idiopathic LIP and idiopathic pleuroparenchymal fibroelastosis (PPFE) into the category of rare IIPs. Additionally, two entities with uncertain clinical and histological features were recognized but excluded from IIPs: Acute fibrinous organizing pneumonia (AFOP) and bronchiolocentric interstitial pneumonia (BIP).[2]

PATHOPHYSIOLOGY

The diverse etiologies of ILDs lead to a spectrum of pathophysiologic changes. Fibrotic involvement of the lung parenchyma, inflammatory/immune infiltration of the interstitium, alveoli, airways, and pulmonary vascular involvement (e.g. in CTD-ILDs like scleroderma) contribute to disturbances in the gaseous exchange, architectural distortion, and recurrent secondary infections.

Clinical Course

The clinical course of ILDs varies depending on the specific type and severity. The clinical course of interstitial lung diseases (ILDs) can vary significantly, ranging from a chronic, slowly progressing condition to rapid deterioration in symptoms, pulmonary function, and imaging findings. This rapid decline is termed progressive pulmonary fibrosis (PPF) and can occur in various ILDs, not just IPF. Additionally, acute exacerbations, similar to those seen in IPF, are also observed in other ILDs, including CTD-ILDs.[3] However, the progression of the disease often leads to hypoxic respiratory failure, pulmonary hypertension, right heart failure, and recurrent secondary infections.

Interstitial lung diseases (ILDs) exhibit diverse clinical courses, ranging from chronic and stable to rapidly progressive, with significant deterioration in symptoms, lung function, and imaging findings.

MANAGEMENT OF INTERSTITIAL LUNG DISEASES

Management of interstitial lung diseases (ILDs) presents a significant challenge due to the limited availability of robust randomized controlled trials. Consequently, treatment strategies rely heavily on institutional expertise and consensus recommendations.

Corticosteroids

For ILDs with prominent inflammatory and autoimmune components, corticosteroids remain a cornerstone of therapy, targeting organ injury through their immunomodulatory effects. Methylprednisolone, prednisone, dexamethasone, and hydrocortisone are the most common agents, employed in both parenteral and oral forms. Two main dosing strategies exist pulse therapy with high doses for short-term control of acute exacerbations and long-term low-dose maintenance therapy for chronic disease control with minimal side effects. Methylprednisolone is frequently used for pulse therapy, and dexamethasone is also a good alternative because of its prolonged action, high glucocorticoid activity (when compared to prednisone), and low mineralocorticoid activity.[4] Beyond the traditional oral and parenteral routes, localized delivery of corticosteroids can be employed in specific scenarios. Intrapleural administration is a valuable option for managing rheumatoid pleural effusions, while intra-articular injections offer targeted relief in cases with joint involvement. Inhaled corticosteroids, although not the first-line therapy for most ILDs, may be considered for patients with bronchiolitis-interstitial patterns or those with superimposed airway inflammation.

The choice of a specific corticosteroid regimen, including dosage, duration, and tapering schedule, requires careful individualization based on the underlying ILD subtype, disease severity, and potential for adverse effects. Balancing the potential benefits of corticosteroids against their well-documented side effects necessitates close monitoring and ongoing reassessment of therapy.

Beyond corticosteroids, a range of other treatment modalities are employed in the ILD armamentarium, depending on the specific disease subtype and individual patient profile. These include immunosuppressive agents, antifibrotic drugs, oxygen therapy, and pulmonary rehabilitation. The optimal treatment plan often involves a multi-pronged approach, combining multiple modalities to address the various facets of the disease and optimize patient outcomes.

Pulse Steroids in ILDs

Pulse steroid therapy, characterized by the administration of supraphysiological doses over a short period, aims to achieve rapid immunomodulation and symptom control in ILDs while minimizing side effects. Traditionally, doses exceeding 250 mg/day of prednisone or equivalent were considered as pulse therapy. However, methylprednisolone has emerged as the preferred agent in recent practice. The Japanese guidelines for acute exacerbation of ILD recommend a pulse therapy regimen of 1 g/day methylprednisolone for 3 days, followed by 1–4 doses weekly, depending on clinical response. Following the pulse, a maintenance dose of 0.5–1 mg/kg/day is administered for 2–4 weeks, followed by gradual tapering in 5 mg dose reductions every 2–4 weeks.[5] Studies suggest that early steroid tapering (>10% decrease within 2 weeks of admission) in acute exacerbations is associated with improved mortality rates.[6]

Interestingly, the initial dose of steroids in acute exacerbations of IPF may influence the risk of recurrence. A study by Ryo Yamazaki suggests that higher initial doses are linked to lower recurrence rates compared to lower doses.[7] This finding underscores the potential importance of tailoring pulse steroid therapy to individual patient needs and disease severity.

Despite the lack of robust randomized controlled trials, pulse steroids have emerged as a valuable therapeutic option in ILDs. A systematic review and meta-analysis revealed no significant association with severe adverse events or overall adverse event rates, further supporting their safety and efficacy.[8] The therapeutic effects of steroids can be categorized as genomic or non-genomic. In the context of pulse therapy, non-genomic actions are believed to play a predominant role due to the rapid onset of action, which cannot be fully explained by classic genomic mechanisms involving gene transcription and protein synthesis.

IDIOPATHIC PULMONARY FIBROSIS (IPF)

The management of idiopathic pulmonary fibrosis (IPF) has undergone significant transformations over the years, particularly regarding the use of corticosteroids. The story of steroid use in idiopathic pulmonary fibrosis (IPF) is a fascinating one, mirroring our evolving understanding of the pathology of this complex disease. Early descriptions of IPF, like "Acute Interstitial Pneumonia" by Hamman and Rich in 1935, paved the way for investigation into its pathology.[9] With the advent of cortisone in 1948, the possibility of treating IPF with steroids arose.[10]

The history of steroid use in IPF treatment dates back to the 1950s when the disease was still known as "Cryptogenic Fibrosing Alveolitis." The rationale for using steroids stemmed from the belief that they could suppress the inflammatory component of the disease and potentially inhibit fibroblast proliferation or offer palliation. By the 1970s and 80s, prednisone dosages were established, and it became a standard therapy for some IPF patients.

The 1999 BTS guidelines for diffuse parenchymal lung diseases (DPLDs) recommended prednisone alone or in combination with azathioprine or cyclophosphamide, with tapering after one month.[11] However, the exact timing for starting steroids remained unclear, and combination therapy (steroids and either azathioprine or cyclophosphamide) was suggested for patients with clinical, physiological, or lung function decline. While benefits were observed in some studies, the low quality of evidence and long-term steroid-associated morbidity raised concerns.[12–14] The 2000 ATS consensus statement further refined these recommendations, reserving this combination therapy for appropriate patients lacking significant comorbidities like obesity or cardiac illness.[15]

Despite frequent use, steroid treatment in this era lacked standardization, with doses ranging from 0.5 to 1 mg/kg/day for 6–8 weeks, followed by tapering to 5–10 mg/day. A study in mild-to-moderate IPF found steroids, alone or in combination with colchicine or cyclophosphamide, failed to prevent disease progression even in the early stages (Fiorucci et al, 2000). While another study showed colchicine offered a safer alternative to steroids, its efficacy was comparable to no therapy at all.[16,17]

ATS 2011 guidelines abandoned steroid monotherapy due to the lack of definitive impact on mortality and the potential for adverse effects.[18] This shift was further solidified by the PANTHER trial, where the combination of steroids, azathioprine, and N-acetylcysteine not only failed to improve outcomes but demonstrated increased mortality compared to the placebo.[19]

As our understanding of ILD pathogenesis evolved, particularly the roles of epithelial-myofibroblast transformation, dysregulated repair mechanisms, and collagen deposition, with minimal involvement of inflammation and immune activation, the reliance on corticosteroids diminished. The emergence of potent antifibrotic agents like pirfenidone and nintedanib, demonstrably slowing disease progression in RCTs, has effectively relegated steroids to a backseat role. Although no randomized controlled trials exist, corticosteroids still hold a role in managing acute exacerbations due to their rapid anti-inflammatory effects. The 2015 ATS IPF treatment guideline and a 2010 Cochrane review echo this position, highlighting the lack of strong evidence for steroids in IPF management.[20,21] Two Bayesian Network Meta-analyses (NMA) published in 2016 and 2017 further contributed to the decline of steroid use in IPF. The 2016 NMA, including the PANTHER trial data, concluded that triple therapy with steroids increased the risk of adverse events without demonstrable benefit. Nintedanib, pirfenidone, and sildenafil were found to offer mortality advantages over steroids.[22,23]

NONSPECIFIC INTERSTITIAL PNEUMONIA (NSIP)

Nonspecific interstitial pneumonia (NSIP) is a type of ILD characterized by lymphocytic inflammation and variable degrees of fibrosis within the lung tissue. Initially coined in

1994 to describe lung biopsy samples lacking specific patterns like UIP or OP/RBILD, the concept of NSIP has evolved.[24] While initially proposed as a provisional diagnosis, the 2002 ATS recommendations and subsequent NSIP workshop established it as a distinct entity.[25]

However, the histological pattern can also occur in association with connective tissue diseases, hypersensitivity pneumonitis, drug-induced lung disease, and infections. Therefore, a thorough workup is crucial to rule out these potential causes and define idiopathic NSIP, where clinical NSIP implies all other etiologies have been excluded.[26]

NSIP's hallmark lies in its temporal homogeneity, characterized by mononuclear cell infiltration of the interstitium and varying degrees of fibrosis. This histopathological spectrum categorizes NSIP into cellular (dominated by inflammation) and fibrotic (dominated by scarring) subtypes. Diagnosis relies on tissue obtained through transbronchial cryo biopsy or surgical biopsy, but the NSIP pattern can co-exist with other distinct entities like UIP, organizing pneumonia, and hypersensitivity pneumonitis.[27]

Treatment

Identifying the underlying cause of NSIP is paramount for optimal management. For instance, hypersensitivity pneumonitis necessitates exposure prevention, while autoimmune diseases may benefit from immunosuppression, and HIV-associated NSIP often responds well to HAART therapy. This individualized approach highlights the importance of accurate diagnosis and underscores the evolution of NSIP from a mere "nonspecific pattern" to a specific entity with diverse etiologies and management strategies (Fig. 5.1).

NSIP treatment involves corticosteroids as the mainstay, with an initial dose of 0.5–1 mg/kg/day prednisolone for a month, followed by gradual tapering over 6–9 months. Steroid-sparing agents like azathioprine or mycophenolate mofetil may be added based on individual needs. Acute cases with rapid respiratory failure may

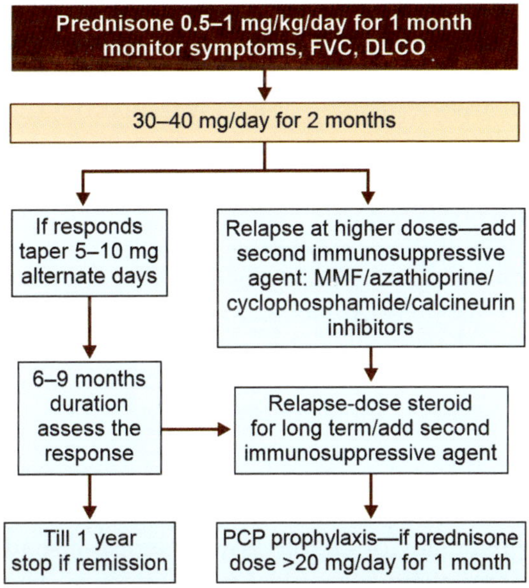

Fig. 5.1: Plan of steroids in NSIP[28]

benefit from pulse therapy with methylprednisolone 1 g/day for 3 days, followed by 1 mg/kg/day for 4 weeks, with further tapering recommended.[28] The lack of randomized controlled trials necessitates highly individualized treatment plans. Symptom scores and pulmonary functions FVC, and DLCO are useful to monitor the disease progression. Regular monitoring after 3 and 6–12 months of NSIP therapy is crucial for assessing disease response and guiding treatment decisions. Non-responders may benefit from additional immunosuppression, like cyclophosphamide, azathioprine, or even colchicine (in specific cases), to avoid unnecessary steroid side effects. Steroid-dependent patients can also consider adding immunosuppressants.

While some studies like Watanabe's show high steroid response rates, Yeon Lee's study highlights risks of higher relapse and mortality with low initial doses or early withdrawal. NSIP generally has an excellent prognosis, with studies like Cho's demonstrating 5-year and 10-year survival rates exceeding 90%. Interestingly, Kondoh's study demonstrated improvement in two-thirds of NSIP patients treated with a combination of pulse steroids, cyclophosphamide, and long-term steroids, contrasting with worse outcomes in IPF patients. Steroid responsiveness in NSIP may be associated with the presence of organizing pneumonia patterns.[29–33]

Prognosis in NSIP is influenced by baseline histopathology, with fibrotic patterns indicating a poorer outlook. Additionally, declining lung function measurements, such as FVC and DLCO, serve as important prognostic markers for disease progression. In conclusion, corticosteroids remain the cornerstone of NSIP treatment, but a comprehensive workup for underlying etiologies is crucial. Identifying and eliminating potential triggers, such as drugs or systemic diseases, can significantly impact prognosis.

ORGANIZING PNEUMONIA (OP)

Organizing pneumonia (OP) is a nonspecific inflammatory reaction primarily affecting the distal airways, triggered by a diverse range of identifiable and unknown causes. It is characterized by distinctive pathological features: plugs of granulation tissue within alveolar ducts and alveoli leading to characteristic nodules and consolidation patches scattered in subpleural areas and along bronchovascular bundles. While "cryptogenic OP" refers to cases with no identifiable cause, other common culprits include post-infectious insults, inhalational injuries, connective tissue diseases, malignancies, and aspiration.

The clinical course exhibits diverse patterns, ranging from spontaneous resolution to remission with steroids and potential relapses. Spontaneous resolution, documented in 3.6% of cases, may be associated with low CRP levels, higher lymphocyte counts, and longer symptom duration before diagnosis. Studies report full resolution rates ranging from 40 to 100%. Clinical variants like acute fulminant forms, cicatricial variants, and unifocal presentations further complicate the picture.[34]

Treatment

While randomized controlled trials are lacking, consensus guidelines advocate corticosteroids as the mainstay of OP therapy. The response to steroids is generally excellent, with around 60% achieving good clinical outcomes. However, resistant forms are observed, particularly in acute fulminant forms and those with fibrotic involvement.

Prednisolone at 1–1.5 mg/kg/day has demonstrated efficacy in resolving symptoms for most patients with organizing pneumonia (OP). For severe cases with respiratory failure, pulsed intravenous methylprednisolone 500–1000 mg/day for 3 days, followed by oral prednisolone 20 mg/day for 3 months with tapering attempts, is often employed. Treatment duration typically extends to 4–6 months, and occasionally up to a year.[34] Despite initial response, a relapse rate of 31.5% has been observed in patients receiving steroids. Prolonged steroid therapy beyond a year did not show significant benefit in reducing relapse rates. Delayed treatment beyond 2 months after symptom onset has also been linked to increased relapse risk. Extensive consolidation and recognizable bronchiectasis on imaging suggest a poorer response to steroids. Balancing the benefits and side effects of corticosteroids is crucial.

Studies suggest that combining clarithromycin with steroids can achieve complete regression in 63% of patients.[35,36] PCP prophylaxis becomes essential for patients receiving high-dose prednisolone of >20 mg/day. Relapses are managed with either low-dose steroids or a combination of steroids and clarithromycin.[37] Rituximab has emerged as a valuable option for steroid-resistant cases.[38] Macrolides, azathioprine, MMF, cyclophosphamide, rituximab, tacrolimus, and intravenous immune globulin (IVIg) represent additional therapeutic avenues in this complex disease.

Post-Covid Organizing Pneumonia

The COVID-19 pandemic's legacy includes a spectrum of post-acute sequelae, with persistent respiratory symptoms and multisystemic manifestations forming the core of "post-COVID syndrome." Within this constellation, organizing pneumonia (OP) emerges as a potential cause, particularly in individuals exhibiting ongoing respiratory complaints and radiological findings suggestive of consolidation. Myall's study reported an incidence of 4.8%, highlighting the potential burden of post-COVID OP.[39] While individual case reports and case series provide valuable insights, early screening at 3 weeks after symptom onset, following exclusion of pulmonary embolism, is crucial for timely diagnosis and intervention in post-COVID patients with persistent respiratory symptoms.

Treatment

Steroids remain the cornerstone in managing post-COVID organizing pneumonia (OP), demonstrating encouraging outcomes across studies. Treatment duration typically varies from 3 to 6 weeks, with both high-dose (40 mg prednisone) and low-dose regimens demonstrating similar effectiveness in reducing symptoms and radiological resolution.[39] Lung function parameters like FVC and DLCO showcased significant improvements of 9.6% and 31.6%, respectively, following steroid therapy. Mycophenolate and clarithromycin were used with good results in those who did not respond to steroids. Interestingly, even post-COVID pulmonary fibrosis (PCPF) patients had shown favorable responses to steroid therapy.[40]

Acute Fibrinous Organizing Pneumonia (AFOP)

Acute fibrinous organizing pneumonia (AFOP) emerged as a distinct histologic entity in 2002, described by Beasley.[41] While initially considered a variant of the diffuse alveolar damage (DAD) pattern, AFOP stands apart due to its characteristic presence of excessive fibrin balls within alveolar ducts and alveoli. Its etiology can be cryptogenic, with no identifiable cause, or secondary to various underlying conditions, including connective tissue diseases and hematological malignancies.[41] Recognizing its unique characteristics, the 2013 ATS classification categorized AFOP as a rare interstitial lung disease (IIP).[42]

Corticosteroids remain the cornerstone of AFOP therapy, demonstrating efficacy in many cases. However, the literature presents a patchwork of case reports exploring alternative approaches like pulse therapy and additional immunosuppressants, with varying outcomes. This highlights the need for further research to optimize management strategies for this complex and relatively new entity.

LYMPHOCYTIC INTERSTITIAL PNEUMONIA (LIP)

Lymphocytic interstitial pneumonia (LIP) is a rare interstitial lung disease (ILD) characterized by the infiltration of lymphocytes into the lung interstitium and alveoli. Despite diverse etiologies, it was reclassified as a rare IIP in the 2013 ATS guidelines. Immunocompromised individuals, including those with HIV infection, congenital immunodeficiency, and autoimmune diseases like Sjögren syndrome, are particularly susceptible to LIP development. However, in some cases, the cause remains unknown, leading to the diagnosis of idiopathic LIP. Precise identification of the underlying etiology is crucial for optimal management. For instance, HIV-associated LIP often responds favorably to antiretroviral therapy (ART), highlighting the importance of targeted interventions based on the causative factor.

Granulomatous Lymphocytic Interstitial Pneumonia (GLILD)

Common variable immunodeficiency (CVID) is one of the most prevalent primary immunodeficiency disorders, characterized by a spectrum of complications due to impaired immune function. Beyond autoimmune, autoinflammatory, infectious, and malignant manifestations, CVID can also present with interstitial lung disease (ILD), affecting 5–15% of cases.[42] Granulomatous lymphocytic interstitial pneumonia (GLILD) is the most common ILD subtype, occurring in 10–30% of CVID patients.[43] Associated lymphadenopathy and splenomegaly can offer diagnostic clues for ILD in this population.[43] Regular monitoring of pulmonary function through spirometry and DLCO is crucial, as worsening clinical status or lung function decline may necessitate medical intervention.

The British Lung Foundation/UK Immunodeficiency Network Consensus Statement defines ILD in CVID as "a distinct clinic radiopathological entity with a lymphocytic infiltrate and/or granuloma in the lungs, occurring in patients where other conditions have been excluded".[44] This consensus establishes corticosteroids as the cornerstone of therapy, emphasizing the importance of optimizing intravenous immunoglobulin (IVIg) before initiating GLILD treatment.[44]

Histopathological analysis with immune cell identification can guide targeted therapy decisions, potentially involving T cell or B cell-specific approaches. A study by Bas Smits reported that 42% of GLILD patients treated with 0.3 mg/kg equivalent prednisone achieved long-term remission and showed improvement in both HRCT scores and pulmonary function.[45]

Sjögren's Syndrome

Sjögren's syndrome, a rare systemic autoimmune disease with exocrine gland dysfunction and lymphocytic hyperactivity, carries a significant risk of interstitial lung disease (ILD). A reported prevalence of 18.8% emphasizes the importance of ILD assessment in Sjögren's patients.[46]

Lymphocytic interstitial pneumonia (LIP) manifests in Sjögren's syndrome with characteristic diffuse ground-glass opacities and cystic lesions. Ground-glass opacities suggest active inflammation, making them potentially responsive to corticosteroids. Notably, a study by Xin Dong showed favourable outcomes with steroids in patients exhibiting dominant ground-glass opacities, while cystic components responded better to cyclophosphamide.[47]

HIV LIP

LIP is also observed in HIV patients, with antiretroviral therapy (ART) serving as the first-line treatment. However, in refractory cases, corticosteroids may be cautiously considered despite potential immune suppression.[48]

Idiopathic LIP

Idiopathic LIP (iLIP) remains a rare entity with an unpredictable course and limited understanding. While corticosteroids are the mainstay of therapy due to frequent steroid responsiveness, the response can be unpredictable.[49] Asymptomatic iLIP cases can be monitored with pulmonary function tests, and any deterioration can prompt steroid initiation. Prednisone at 1 mg/kg/day for 8–12 weeks, followed by tapering, is a common regimen with a typical treatment duration of 6–12 months. Azathioprine and mycophenolate mofetil (MMF) may be employed to minimize steroid dosage.[50] Unfortunately, the 5-year mortality rate for iLIP remains high, ranging from 33 to 50%.[50]

ACUTE INTERSTITIAL PNEUMONIA (AIP)

Acute interstitial pneumonia (AIP), a rare and fulminant type of interstitial lung disease (ILD), presents with rapidly progressive hypoxic respiratory failure and carries a high mortality rate exceeding 50%.[1] Histologically, AIP manifests as diffuse alveolar damage (DAD), mirroring the pattern observed in acute respiratory distress syndrome (ARDS).

Despite the absence of definitive therapy established through randomized controlled trials (RCTs), corticosteroids remain the mainstay of treatment in AIP. Pulse therapy with methylprednisolone at 0.5–1 g/day for 3 days, followed by tapering oral prednisolone, is often employed. However, optimal dosing and treatment duration require individualization based on response and tolerance. Due to the poor prognosis associated with AIP, lung transplantation may be considered in select cases with limited response to conventional therapy.

DIP/RBILD

Desquamative interstitial pneumonia (DIP) and respiratory bronchiolitis-interstitial lung disease (RB-ILD) are rare forms of idiopathic interstitial pneumonia (IIP) with a strong association with smoking.[1] While the 2013 ATS guidelines categorized them as ILDs of known causes, it is important to note that DIP can occur in other settings, albeit less frequently (around 20%).[51] The term "desquamative" in DIP is a historical misnomer, as the alveoli lack desquamated cells. Instead, the hallmark features are accumulated pigmented macrophages within the alveoli, often accompanied by inflammatory cells and varying degrees of interstitial fibrosis.[51] RBILD, on the other hand, is characterized by inflammation and the accumulation of yellow-brown macrophages within the respiratory bronchioles and alveolar spaces. Clinically, radiologically, and in terms of pulmonary function, DIP and RBILD present with significant overlap, making differentiation challenging.

Treatment

Smoking cessation remains the cornerstone of therapy for DIP and RB-ILD. Studies, including one by Nakanishi, have shown significant improvement in symptoms, HRCT findings, and DLCO following smoking cessation.[52] These changes, including the resolution of centrilobular nodules and GGO, correspond to improvements in the underlying respiratory bronchiolitis. In cases with mild to moderate disease, smoking cessation and follow-up can often lead to clinical benefit.

However, in patients with persistent symptoms, hypoxia, progressive functional impairment, or those who fail to respond to smoking cessation alone, a trial of corticosteroids may be warranted. Prednisolone doses ranging from 0.5 to 1 mg/kg/day for 6–8 weeks, followed by tapering to 5–10 mg, are commonly employed. Interestingly, studies like Ryu et al reported a better therapeutic response to steroids in RB-ILD compared to DIP, with improvements in symptoms, pulmonary function, and imaging, but relapse often occurs upon cessation of therapy.[53] Other studies, such as Joshua Portnoy's, have not demonstrated significant improvement in symptoms or physiological parameters with either steroids or immunosuppressants.[53]

ACUTE EXACERBATIONS OF INTERSTITIAL LUNG DISEASES (AE-ILD)

Fibrotic interstitial lung diseases (ILDs) typically progress gradually, but some patients experience rapid clinical decline and physiological compromise. Addressing this need, the 2007 ATS guidelines defined acute exacerbations of idiopathic pulmonary fibrosis (IPF) as sudden, unexplained deterioration in patients with established IPF.[54] This concept extends beyond IPF, observed in other ILDs like connective tissue disease-associated ILD and hypersensitivity pneumonitis.

A refined definition emerged in 2016, characterizing acute exacerbation of IPF as a clinically significant deterioration with newly developed diffuse alveolar abnormalities.[4] Revised diagnostic criteria include acute worsening or development dyspnea typically <1 month duration, new radiological worsening associated with ground glassing or consolidation in the background of UIP pattern, background IPF diagnosis, and exclusion of causes like cardiac failure or fluid overload. Based on how well these criteria are met, the exacerbation is classified as acute exacerbation (AE), suspected AE group, or AE of known cause group. Interestingly, steroid requirements did not differ significantly between these groups.[54]

Management Challenges

Fibrotic interstitial lung diseases (ILDs) experience an average of 4.1 acute exacerbations per 100 patient-years, contributing to 50% of hospital mortality.[4] These exacerbations can be idiopathic or triggered by infections, surgery, etc., and pose a significant management challenge. While no randomized controlled trials exist for steroid use in exacerbations, several cohort studies and anecdotal reports suggest potential benefits. Japanese guidelines recommend pulse methylprednisolone (1 g/kg/day for 3 days, followed by weekly tapering based on response).[9] Oda Keishi's study demonstrated an improved prognosis with co-trimoxazole and macrolides alongside high-dose steroid.[55] Although no definitive evidence exists, uncontrolled cohort studies offer insights. Suzuki's study (2011) reported favorable outcomes with pulse steroids and rapid tapering,[56] while Anan et al (2015) observed low mortality with early steroid tapering and higher initial doses associated with lower recurrence.[57,58] Similarly, Toru Ari (2017) found high-dose prednisone (>0.6 mg/kg/day) to be prognostically favorable.[59] Finally, YONATAN EDEL's meta-analysis suggests pulse steroids as a safe approach.[60]

Various immunosuppressive agents have been explored, including cyclophosphamide, tacrolimus, cyclosporine, rituximab, polymyxin B hemoperfusion (PMX), and even thrombomodulin IV and IVIg.[61,62] While a case series suggests improved survival with pulse steroids combined with cyclophosphamide,[63] larger studies like EXAFIP using IV cyclophosphamide unfortunately showed increased 3-month mortality.[64] A study comparing acute exacerbations (AEs) in idiopathic pulmonary fibrosis (IPF) and non-IPF interstitial lung diseases (ILDs) (including NSIP, hypersensitivity pneumonitis, CTD-ILD, and sarcoidosis) revealed interesting findings. While both groups shared similar outcomes, patients with non-IPF AEs experienced a longer time to their first AE and had worse outcomes if their underlying disease was more severe at baseline.[65] This study, based on the 2016 diagnostic criteria, observed that 90% of patients received pulse therapy with 500–1000 mg methylprednisolone alongside antibiotics and other immunosuppressants, followed by steroid tapering. Another study echoed these findings, reporting similar mortality rates in both AE-IPF and AE-non-IPF groups, with 71% of patients receiving high-dose steroids.[66]

Recent studies on acute exacerbations (AEs) in systemic autoimmune ILDs showed an estimated incidence of around 5.77 AEs per 100 patients annually.[67] Interestingly, the frequency of exacerbations appears similar between IPF and CTD-ILD patients, but the prognosis seems more favorable in the CTD-ILD group.[68] Treatment options commonly include methylprednisolone, IVIg, IV cyclophosphamide, and rituximab.[69] While studies suggest a potential survival benefit with rituximab, larger trials are needed to confirm statistical significance. A recent study by Enomoto (2022) identified rheumatoid arthritis, mixed connective tissue disease (MCTD), and systemic sclerosis (SSc) as the most common autoimmune culprits in AE development.[70] Furthermore, this study found that adding cyclophosphamide to the treatment regimen did not improve overall prognosis.

Despite the significant burden of acute exacerbations in both idiopathic pulmonary fibrosis (IPF) and non-IPF interstitial lung diseases (ILDs), no established guidelines currently dictate their management. Treatment remains largely driven by anecdotal experience, with pulse steroids often serving as the first line of defense. While high-dose prednisolone (>0.6 mg/kg/day) with rapid tapering is often employed, the addition of other immunosuppressants has yielded inconsistent results across different studies. Unfortunately, mortality remains high, highlighting the need for further research and more definitive treatment approaches.

PROGRESSIVE PULMONARY FIBROSIS (PPF)

Progressive pulmonary fibrosis (PPF), distinct from idiopathic pulmonary fibrosis (IPF), encompasses a complex spectrum of interstitial lung diseases (ILDs) with progressive lung fibrosis. Diagnosed in patients with radiological evidence of fibrosis and at least two of three criteria within a year-worsening symptoms, declining pulmonary function (FVC drop >5% or DLCO >10%), or radiological worsening—without alternative explanations.

Encompassing various ILDs like fibrotic nonspecific interstitial pneumonia, unclassifiable ILDs, CTD-associated ILDs, and occupational exposure-related ILDs, PPF exhibits a wider range of etiologies than IPF.[71] Its prevalence, estimated at 6.9–70.3 per 100,000 individuals, highlights the significant burden of this entity. For PPF patients progressing despite standard therapy, nintedanib has emerged as a potential treatment option. However, the uncontrolled, self-perpetuating nature of PPF fibrosis suggests a limited role for corticosteroids in standard management. Further research is crucial to better characterize this complex entity and refine therapeutic strategies.

INTERSTITIAL PNEUMONIA WITH AUTOIMMUNE FEATURES (IPAF)

Interstitial pneumonia with autoimmune features (IPAF) marks a distinct entity within the spectrum of interstitial lung disease (ILD). It encompasses individuals exhibiting both ILD and a combination of clinical, serologic, and/or pulmonary morphologic features suggestive of an underlying systemic autoimmune condition but does not meet current rheumatologic criteria for a characterized.[5] The definition includes clinical, serological, and morphological domains to fit into this group allowing for monitoring and clinical response. The prevalence of IPAF within the ILD population is estimated at 7.3% , and studies like John K. Macintosh's suggest a potential progression to clinically recognizable CTD in 10–20% of IPAF cases over time.[6] Understanding and managing IPAF remains an active area of research, intending to improve diagnosis, predict CTD evolution, and optimise treatment strategies for this complex group of patients.

Management of IPAF remains a complex and evolving area, reflecting the diverse and incompletely understood nature of this entity. However, the presence of autoimmune features suggests a rationale for immunosuppressive therapy. CTD-ILD management principles often guide treatment, with steroids, cyclophosphamide, mycophenolate mofetil (MMF), azathioprine, and rituximab being commonly employed. A retrospective analysis revealed promising outcomes with steroid use in 82% of IPAF patients, with no mortality observed.[72]

Respiratory impairment, affecting nearly half of IPAF patients and often presenting early in the disease course, underscores the significant clinical burden.[73] Intriguingly, treatment efficacy appears to differ based on IPAF patterns. Systemic glucocorticosteroids and rituximab show promising outcomes in UIP patterns, suggesting distinct pathogenic mechanisms compared to classical IPF and CTD-ILDs.[73] Similarly, for NSIP patterns, cyclosporine/tacrolimus demonstrates superior efficacy compared to MMF and azathioprine.[73] This pattern-specific response is further supported by evidence suggesting better overall outcomes with immunosuppressive therapy compared to antifibrotic agents in IPAF.[74] These findings highlight the importance of considering disease patterns when tailoring treatment strategies for IPAF patients, with personalized approaches holding the potential to optimize outcomes and improve the management of this complex entity.

REFERENCES

1. American Thoracic Society. International Multidisciplinary Consensus Classification of the Idiopathic Interstitial Pneumonias. This joint statement of the American Thoracic Society (ATS), and the European Respiratory Society (ERS) was adopted by the ATS board of directors, in June 2001 and by the ERS Executive Committee, in 2001. Am J Respir Crit Care Med, 2002;165:277–304.
2. Travis WD, Costabel U, Hansell DM, King Jr TE, Lynch DA, Nicholson AG, Ryerson CJ, Ryu JH, Selman M, Wells AU, Behr J. An official American Thoracic Society/European Respiratory Society statement: update of the international multidisciplinary classification of the idiopathic interstitial pneumonia. American journal of respiratory and critical care medicine. 2013 15;188(6):733–48.
3. Raghu G, Remy-Jardin M, Richeldi L, Thomson CC, Inoue Y, Johkoh T, Kreuter M, Lynch DA, Maher TM, Martinez FJ, Molina-Molina M. Idiopathic pulmonary fibrosis (an update) and progressive pulmonary fibrosis in adults: an official ATS/ERS/JRS/ALAT clinical practice guideline. American *Journal of Respiratory and Critical Care Medicine*. 2022 1;205(9): e18–47.
4. Sinha A, Bagga A. Pulse steroid therapy. The Indian Journal of Pediatrics. 2008;75:1057–66.
5. Homma S, Bando M, Azuma A, Sakamoto S, Sugino K, Ishii Y, Izumi S, Inase N, Inoue Y, Ebina M, Ogura T. Japanese guideline for the treatment of idiopathic pulmonary fibrosis. Respiratory investigation. 2018 1;56(4):268–91.
6. Anan K, Kataoka Y, Ichikado K, et al. Early corticosteroid dose tapering in patients with acute exacerbation of idiopathic pulmonary fibrosis. Respir Res 24, 107 (2023). https://doi.org/10.1186/s12931-023-02411-8.
7. Yamazaki R, Nishiyama O, Saeki S, Sano H, Iwanaga T, Tohda Y. Initial therapeutic dose of corticosteroid for an acute exacerbation of IPF is associated with subsequent early recurrence of another exacerbation. Scientific Reports. 2021 11;11(1):5782.
8. Edel Y, Avni T, Shepshelovich D, Reich S, Rozen-Zvi B, Elbaz M, Leibovici L, Molad Y, Gafter- Gvili A. The safety of pulse corticosteroid therapy- systematic review and meta-analysis. InSeminars in Arthritis and Rheumatism 2020 1 (Vol. 50, No. 3, pp. 534–45). WB Saunders.
9. Homolka J. Idiopathic pulmonary fibrosis: a historical review. CMAJ: Canadian Medical Association Journal. 1987 12;137(11):1003.mapel.
10. Mapel DW, Samet JM, Coultas DB. Corticosteroids and the treatment of idiopathic pulmonary fibrosis: past, present, and future. Chest. 1996 1;110(4):1058–67.
11. SOCIETY BT, Committee SO. The diagnosis, assessment and treatment of diffuse parenchymal lung disease in adults. Thorax. 1999;54(Suppl 1):S1.
12. Johnson MA, Kwan S, Snell NJ, Nunn AJ, Darbyshire JH, Turner-Warwick M. Randomised controlled trial comparing prednisolone alone with cyclophosphamide and low dose prednisolone in combination in cryptogenic fibrosing alveolitis. Thorax. 1989 1;44(4):280–8.
13. Raghu G, Depaso WJ, Cain K, Hammar SP, Wetzel CE, Dreis DF, Hutchinson J, Pardee NE, Winterbauer RH. Azathioprine combined with prednisone in the treatment of idiopathic pulmonary fibrosis: a prospective double-blind, randomized, placebo-controlled clinical trial. Am Rev Respir Dis.1991 1;144(2):291–6.
14. Kondoh Y, Taniguchi H, Yokoi T, Nishiyama O, Ohishi T, Kato T, Suzuki K, Suzuki R. Cyclophosphamide and low-dose prednisolone in idiopathic pulmonary fibrosis and fibrosing nonspecific interstitial pneumonia. European Respiratory Journal. 2005 Mar 1;25(3):528–33.
15. American Thoracic Society. Idiopathic pulmonary fibrosis: diagnosis and treatment. International consensus statement. American Thoracic Society (ATS), and the European Respiratory Society (ERS). Am J Respir Crit Care Med. 2000(161):646–64.

16. Fiorucci F, Lucantoni G, Paone G, Zotti M, Li Bianchi E, Serpilli M, Regiment P, Cammarella I, Puglisi G, Schmid G. Colchicine, cyclophosphamide and prednisone in the treatment of mild-moderate idiopathic pulmonary fibrosis: comparison of three currently available therapeutic regimens. European review for medical and pharmacological sciences. 2008 1;12(2):105.
17. Douglas WW, Ryu JH, Swensen SJ, Offord KP, Schroeder DR, Caron GM, DeREMEE RA, Lung Study Group*. Colchicine versus prednisone in the treatment of idiopathic pulmonary fibrosis: a randomized prospective study. *American Journal of respiratory and critical care medicine*. 1998 1;158(1):220–5.
18. Raghu G, Collard HR, Egan JJ, Martinez FJ, Behr J, Brown KK, Colby TV, Cordier JF, Flaherty KR, Lasky JA, Lynch DA. An official ATS/ERS/JRS/ALAT statement: idiopathic pulmonary fibrosis: evidence-based guidelines for diagnosis and management. *American Journal of respiratory and critical care medicine*. 2011 Mar 15;183(6):788–824.
19. Idiopathic Pulmonary Fibrosis Clinical Research Network. Prednisone, azathioprine, and N acetylcysteine for pulmonary fibrosis. *New England Journal of Medicine*. 2012 24;366(21):1968–77.
20. Raghu G, Rochwerg B, Zhang Y, Garcia CA, Azuma A, Behr J, Brozek JL, Collard HR, Cunningham W, Homma S, Johkoh T. An official ATS/ERS/JRS/ALAT clinical practice guideline: treatment of idiopathic pulmonary fibrosis. An update of the 2011 clinical practice guideline. American journal of respiratory and critical care medicine. 2015 15;192(2):e3-19.
21. Richeldi L, Davies HRHR, Spagnolo P, Luppi F. Corticosteroids for idiopathic pulmonary fibrosis. Cochrane Database of Systematic Reviews 2003;3(2):34–47.
22. Rochwerg B, Neupane B, Zhang Y, Garcia CC, Raghu G, Richeldi L, Brozek J, Beyene J, Schünemann H. Treatment of idiopathic pulmonary fibrosis: a network meta-analysis. BMC medicine. 2016;14(1):1–2.
23. Fleetwood K, McCool R, Glanville J, Edwards SC, Gsteiger S, Daigl M, Fisher M. Systematic review and network meta-analysis of idiopathic pulmonary fibrosis treatments. *Journal of managed care and speciality pharmacy*. 2017;23(3-b Suppl):S5–16.
24. Katzenstein AL, Fiorelli RF. Nonspecific interstitial pneumonia/fibrosis. Histologic features and clinical significance. The American journal of surgical pathology. 1994 Feb 1;18(2):136–47.
25. Travis WD, Hunninghake G, King Jr TE, Lynch DA, Colby TV, Galvin JR, Brown KK, Chung MP, Cordier JF, Du Bois RM, Flaherty KR. Idiopathic nonspecific interstitial pneumonia: report of an American Thoracic Society project. *American Journal of respiratory and critical care medicine*. 2008 Jun 15;177(12):1338–47.
26. Flaherty KR, Martinez FJ. Nonspecific interstitial pneumonia. InSeminars in respiratory and critical care medicine 2006 Dec (Vol. 27, No. 06, pp. 652–658). Copyright© 2006 by Thieme Medical Publishers, Inc., 333 Seventh Avenue, New York, NY 10001, USA.
27. Tomassetti S, Ryu JH, Piciucchi S, Chilosi M, Poletti V. Nonspecific interstitial pneumonia: what is the optimal approach to management?. InSeminars in respiratory and critical care medicine 2016 Jun (Vol. 37, No. 03, pp. 378–394). Thieme Medical Publishers.
28. Nayfeh AS, Chippa V, Moore DR. Nonspecific Interstitial Pneumonitis. [Updated 2023 Apr 16]. In: StatPearls [Internet]. Treasure Island (FL): StatPearls Publishing; 2023 Jan.
29. Watanabe K, Higuchi K, Ninomiya K, Ohshima T, Aritomi T, Kawabata Y, Yoshida M. Steroid treatment based on the findings of transbronchial biopsy in idiopathic interstitial pneumonia. *European Respiratory Journal*. 2002 Nov 1;20(5):1213–9.
30. Park IN, Jegal Y, Kim DS, Do KH, Yoo B, Shim TS, Lim CM, Lee SD, Koh Y, Kim WS, Kim WD. Clinical course and lung function change of idiopathic nonspecific interstitial pneumonia. *European Respiratory Journal*. 2009 Jan 1;33(1):68–76.
31. Lee JY, Jin SM, Lee BJ, Chung DH, Jang BG, Park HS, Lee SM, Yim JJ, Yang SC, Yoo CG, Han SK. Treatment response and long-term follow-up results of nonspecific interstitial pneumonia. *Journal of Korean Medical Science*. 2012 Jun 1;27(6):661–7.
32. Xu W, Xiao Y, Liu H, Qin M, Zheng W, Shi J. Nonspecific interstitial pneumonia: clinical associations and outcomes. BMC Pulmonary Medicine. 2014 Dec;14(1):1–0.

33. Cho HK, Chung MP, Soo Lee K, Chung MJ, Han J, Kwon OJ, Yoo H. Clinical characteristics and prognostic factors of fibrotic nonspecific interstitial pneumonia. Therapeutic Advances in Respiratory Disease. 2022 Apr;16:17534666221089468.
34. Bradley B, Branley HM, Egan JJ, Greaves MS, Hansell DM, Harrison NK, Hirani N, Hubbard R, Lake F, Millar AB, Wallace WA. Interstitial lung disease guideline: the British Thoracic Society in collaboration with the Thoracic Society of Australia and New Zealand and the Irish Thoracic Society (vol 63, Suppl V, pg v1, 2008). Thorax. 2008 Nov 1;63(11):1029-.
35. Petitpierre N, Cottin V, Marchand-Adam S, Hirschi S, Rigaud D, Court-Fortune I, Jouneau S, Israël-Biet D, Molard A, Cordier JF, Lazor R. A 12-week combination of clarithromycin and prednisone compared to a 24-week prednisone alone treatment in cryptogenic and radiation-induced organizing pneumonia. Sarcoidosis, Vasculitis, and Diffuse Lung Diseases. 2018;35(3):230.
36. Radzikowska E, Wiatr E, Langford R, Bestry I, Skoczylas A, Szczepulska-Wójcik E, Gawryluk D, Rudziński P, Chorostowska-Wynimko J, Roszkowski-Śliż K. Cryptogenic organizing pneumonia—Results of treatment with clarithromycin versus corticosteroids—Observational study. PLoS One. 2017 Sep 25;12(9):e0184739.
37. Radzikowska E, Fijolek J. Update on cryptogenic organizing pneumonia. Frontiers in Medicine. 2023 Apr 20;10:1146782.
38. Shitenberg D, Fruchter O, Fridel L, Kramer MR. Successful rituximab therapy in steroid-resistant, cryptogenic organizing pneumonia: a case series. Respiration. 2015 Aug 1;90(2):155–9.
39. Myall KJ, Mukherjee B, Castanheira AM, Lam JL, Benedetti G, Mak SM, Preston R, Thillai M, Dewar A, Molyneaux PL, West AG. Persistent post–COVID–19 interstitial lung disease. An observational study of corticosteroid treatment. Annals of the American Thoracic Society. 2021 May;18(5):799–806.
40. Fukihara J, Kondoh Y. COVID-19 and interstitial lung diseases: a multifaceted look at the relationship between the two diseases. Respiratory Investigation. 2023 Jun 20.
41. Beasley MB, Franks TJ, Galvin JR, Gochuico B, Travis WD. Acute fibrinous and organizing pneumonia: a histologic pattern of lung injury and possible variant of diffuse alveolar damage. Archives of pathology and laboratory medicine. 2002 Sep 1;126(9):1064–70.
42. Prasse A, Kayser G, Warnatz K. Common variable immunodeficiency-associated granulomatous and interstitial lung disease. Current opinion in pulmonary medicine. 2013 Sep1;19(5):503–9.
43. Rao N, Mackinnon AC, Routes JM. Granulomatous and lymphocytic interstitial lung disease: a spectrum of pulmonary histopathologic lesions in common variable immunodeficiency—histologic and immunohistochemical analyses of 16 cases. Human pathology. 2015 Sep 1;46(9):1306–14.
44. Hurst JR, Verma N, Lowe D, Baxendale HE, Jolles S, Kelleher P, Longhurst HJ, Patel SY, Renzoni EA, Sander CR and Avery GR, 2017. British Lung Foundation/United Kingdom Primary Immunodeficiency Network consensus statement on the definition, diagnosis, and management of granulomatous-lymphocytic interstitial lung disease in common variable immunodeficiency disorders. The Journal of Allergy and Clinical Immunology: In Practice, 5(4), pp. 938–45.
45. Lamers OA, Smits BM, Leavis HL, de Bree GJ, Cunningham-Rundles C, Dalm VA, Ho HE, Hurst JR, IJspeert H, Prevaes SM, Robinson A. Treatment strategies for GLILD in common variable immunodeficiency: a systematic review. Frontiers in Immunology. 2021 Apr 15;12:606099.
46. He SH, He YJ, Guo KJ, Liang X, Li SS, Li TF. Risk factors for progression of interstitial lung disease in Sjögren's syndrome: A single-centered, retrospective study. Clinical Rheumatology. 2022 Apr 1:1–9.
47. Dong X, Gao YL, Lu Y, Zheng Y. Characteristics of primary Sjögren's syndrome-related lymphocytic interstitial pneumonia. Clinical Rheumatology. 2021 Feb;40:601–12.
48. Tasdemir MN, Aslan S. Lymphocytic Interstitial Pneumonia in a Man with Human Immunodeficiency Virus Infection. Revista da Sociedade Brasileira de Medicina Tropical. 2023 Jun 2;56: e0055–2023.
49. Swigris JJ, Berry GJ, Raffin TA, Kuschner WG. Lymphoid interstitial pneumonia: a narrative review. Chest. 2002 Dec 1;122(6):2150–64.
50. Panchabhai TS, Farver C, Highland KB. Lymphocytic interstitial pneumonia. Clinics in Chest Medicine. 2016 Sep 1;37(3):463–74.

51. Ryu JH, Myers JL, Capizzi SA, Douglas WW, Vassallo R, Decker PA. Desquamative interstitial pneumonia and respiratory bronchiolitis-associated interstitial lung disease. Chest. 2005 Jan 1;127(1):178–84.
52. Nakanishi M, Demura Y, Mizuno S, Ameshima S, Chiba Y, Miyamori I, Itoh H, Kitaichi M, Ishizaki T. Changes in HRCT findings in patients with respiratory bronchiolitis-associated interstitial lung disease after smoking cessation. European Respiratory Journal. 2007 Mar 1;29(3):453–61.
53. Portnoy J, Veraldi KL, Schwarz MI, Cool CD, Curran-Everett D, Cherniack RM, King Jr TE, Brown KK. Respiratory bronchiolitis-interstitial lung disease. Chest. 2007 Mar 1;131(3):664–71.
54. Collard HR, Moore BB, Flaherty KR, Brown KK, Kaner RJ, King Jr TE, Lasky JA, Loyd JE, Noth I, Olman MA, Raghu G. Acute exacerbations of idiopathic pulmonary fibrosis. American journal of respiratory and critical care medicine. 2007 Oct 1;176(7):636–43.
55. Oda K, Yatera K, Fujino Y, Ishimoto H, Nakao H, Hanaka T, Ogoshi T, Kido T, Fushimi K, Matsuda S, Mukae H. Efficacy of concurrent treatments in idiopathic pulmonary fibrosis patients with a rapid progression of respiratory failure: an analysis of a national administrative database in Japan. BMC Pulmonary Medicine. 2016 Dec;16(1):1–9.
56. Suzuki H, Sekine Y, Yoshida S, Suzuki M, Shibuya K, Yonemori Y, Hiroshima K, Nakatani Y, Mizuno S, Takiguchi Y, Yoshino I. Risk of acute exacerbation of interstitial pneumonia after pulmonary resection for lung cancer in patients with idiopathic pulmonary fibrosis based on preoperative high- resolution computed tomography. Surgery today. 2011 Jul; 41:914–21.
57. Anan K, Kataoka Y, Ichikawa K, Kawamura K, Johkoh T, Fujimoto K, Tobino K, Tachikawa R, Ito H, Nakamura T, Kishaba T. Early corticosteroid dose tapering in patients with acute exacerbation of idiopathic pulmonary fibrosis. Respiratory Research. 2022 Dec;23(1):1–0.
58. Yamazaki R, Nishiyama O, Saeki S, Sano H, Iwanaga T, Tohda Y. Initial therapeutic dose of corticosteroid for an acute exacerbation of IPF is associated with subsequent early recurrence of another exacerbation. Scientific Reports. 2021 Mar 11;11(1):5782.
59. Arai T, Tachibana K, Sugimoto C, Inoue Y, Tokura S, Okuma T, Akira M, Kitaichi M, Hayashi S, Inoue Y. High-dose prednisolone after intravenous methylprednisolone improves prognosis of acute exacerbation in idiopathic interstitial pneumonias. Respirology. 2017 Oct;22(7):1363–70.
60. Edel Y, Avni T, Shepshelovich D, Reich S, Rozen-Zvi B, Elbaz M, Leibovici L, Molad Y, Gafter- Gvili A. The safety of pulse corticosteroid therapy-Systematic review and meta-analysis. InSeminars in Arthritis and Rheumatism 2020 1;50(3):534–545 (Vol. 50, No. 3, pp. 534-545). WB Saunders.
61. Arai T, Kida H, Ogata Y, Marumo S, Matsuoka H, Gohma I, Yamamoto S, Mori M, Sugimoto C, Tachibana K, Akira M. Efficacy of recombinant thrombomodulin for poor prognostic cases of acute exacerbation in idiopathic interstitial pneumonia: secondary analysis of the SETUP trial. BMJ Open Respiratory Research. 2020 May 1;7(1):e000558.
62. Higo H, Ichikawa H, Nakamura N, Fujii M, Matsuoka K, Seki S, Wada T, Suzaki N, Nagata T, Arakawa Y, Mori Y. Intravenous immunoglobulin for acute exacerbation of fibrotic idiopathic interstitial pneumonia. Sarcoidosis, Vasculitis, and Diffuse Lung Diseases. 2022;39(4).
63. Novelli L, Ruggiero R, De Giacomo F, Biffi A, Faverio P, Bilucaglia L, Gamberini S, Messinesi G, Pesci A. Corticosteroid and cyclophosphamide in acute exacerbation of idiopathic pulmonary fibrosis: a single centre experience and. Sarcoidosis Vasculitis and Diffuse Lung Diseases. 2016; 33:385–91.
64. Naccache JM, Jouneau S, Didier M, Borie R, Cachanado M, Bourdin A, Reynaud-Gaubert M, Bonniaud P, Israël-Biet D, Prévot G, Hirschi S. Cyclophosphamide added to glucocorticoids in acute exacerbation of idiopathic pulmonary fibrosis (EXAFIP): a randomised, double-blind, placebo-controlled, phase 3 trial. The Lancet Respiratory Medicine. 2022 Jan 1;10(1):26–34.
65. Suzuki A, Kondoh Y, Brown KK, Johkoh T, Kataoka K, Fukuoka J, Kimura T, Matsuda T, Yokoyama T, Fukihara J, Ando M. Acute exacerbations of fibrotic interstitial lung diseases. Respirology. 2020 May;25(5):525–34.
66. Faverio P, Stainer A, Conti S, Madotto F, De Giacomi F, Della Zoppa M, Vancheri A, Pellegrino MR, Tonelli R, Cerri S, Clini EM. Differences between Acute Exacerbations of Idiopathic Pulmonary Fibrosis and Other Interstitial Lung Diseases. Diagnostics. 2021 Sep 6;11(9):1623.

67. Andreina Manfredi1Flaherty KR, Wells AU, Cottin V, Devaraj A, Walsh SL, Inoue Y, Richeldi L, Kolb M, Tetzlaff K, Stowasser S, Coeck C. Nintedanib in progressive fibrosing interstitial lung diseases. New England Journal of Medicine. 2019 Oct 31;381(18):1718–27.
68. Cao M, Sheng J, Qiu X, Wang D, Wang D, Wang Y, Xiao Y, Cai H. Acute exacerbations of fibrosing interstitial lung disease associated with connective tissue diseases: a population-based study. BMC Pulmonary Medicine. 2019 Dec;19:1–0.
69. Singh P, Thakur B, Mohapatra AK, Padhan P. Clinical features and outcome of acute exacerbation in connective tissue disease-associated interstitial lung disease: A single-centre study from India. International Journal of Rheumatic Diseases. 2019 Sep;22(9):1741–5.
70. Enomoto N, Naoi H, Mochizuka Y, Isayama T, Tanaka Y, Fukada A, Aono Y, Katsumata M, Yasui H, Mori K, Karayama M. Frequency, the proportion of PF-ILD, and prognostic factors in patients with acute exacerbation of ILD related to systemic autoimmune diseases. BMC Pulmonary Medicine. 2022 Oct 26;22(1):387.
71. Cottin V, Hirani NA, Hotchkin DL, Nambiar AM, Ogura T, Otaola M, Skowasch D, Park JS, Poonyagariyagorn HK, Wuyts W, Wells AU. Presentation, diagnosis and clinical course of the spectrum of progressive-fibrosing interstitial lung diseases. European Respiratory Review. 2018 Dec 31;27(150).
72. Chartrand S, Swigris JJ, Stanchev L, Lee JS, Brown KK, Fischer A. Clinical features and natural history of interstitial pneumonia with autoimmune features: a single centre experience. Respiratory medicine. 2016 Oct 1;119:150–4.
73. Nieto MA, Sanchez-Pernaute O, Vadillo C, Rodriguez-Nieto MJ, Romero-Bueno F, López-Muñiz B, Cebrian L, Rio-Ramirez MT, Laporta R, Bonilla G, Cobo T. Functional respiratory impairment and related factors in patients with interstitial pneumonia with autoimmune features (IPAF): Multicenter study from NEREA registry. Respiratory Research. 2023 Jan 18;24(1):19.
74. Yamano Y, Kataoka K, Takei R, Sasano H, Yokoyama T, Matsuda T, Kimura T, Mori Y, Furukawa T, Fukuoka J, Johko T. Interstitial pneumonia with autoimmune features and histologic usual interstitial pneumonia treated with anti-fibrotic versus immunosuppressive therapy. Respiratory Investigation. 2023 May 1;61(3):297–305.

Chapter

6

Steroids in Sarcoidosis and Hypersensitivity Pneumonitis

G Uma Sri • M Ramakrishna Reddy

INTRODUCTION

Sarcoidosis, a multisystemic disorder of unknown etiology, can lead to organ dysfunction and significantly impact quality of life. Thoracic involvement occurs in 90% of patients, primarily manifesting as bilateral, symmetrical hilar adenopathy. The lungs remain the most frequently affected organ. In sarcoidosis, the hallmark granulomatous inflammation arises from a dysregulated immune response triggered by an unknown environmental factor in individuals with a genetic predisposition. These granulomas are composed primarily of macrophages that transform into epithelioid cells, eventually fusing into multinucleated giants. CD4+ helper T cells reside within the granuloma, while CD8+ T cells, regulatory T cells (Tregs), fibroblasts, and B cells form the surrounding periphery, highlighting the complex interplay of immune cells contributing to this enigmatic disease process.[1] Non-caseating granulomas infiltrate the bronchovascular bundles and interstitium, leading to impaired gas exchange, architectural distortion (e.g. fibrosis), and reduced lung compliance. While many patients, especially those with early-stage (Stage 1) sarcoidosis, remain asymptomatic and are diagnosed incidentally through chest imaging findings, 30–50% experience nonspecific respiratory symptoms. These can include non-productive cough, breathlessness, and chest pain.

TREATMENT OF SARCOIDOSIS

The landmark 1999 guidelines on sarcoidosis diagnosis and management, established by the ERS, ATS, and WASOG, laid the foundation for understanding this complex disease.[2] To update and refine treatment approaches, the ERS Task Force undertook a systematic review of the evidence, culminating in new guidelines for managing pulmonary, cutaneous, cardiac, and neurological manifestations alongside sarcoidosis-associated fatigue (SAF) and small-fibre neuropathy (SFN).[3] This comprehensive review aims to provide clinicians with evidence-based guidance for effectively managing the diverse presentations of sarcoidosis and improving patient outcomes.

The treatment of sarcoidosis depends on the disease severity and extent at diagnosis. Treatment should be individualized for patients with symptomatic sarcoidosis that impacts their quality of life (QOL) or those with lung function decline or increased risk for long-term complications. Relying solely on chest X-rays, scadding stages, or CT scans, especially in the early stages, is discouraged.[4] Asymptomatic individuals with just intrathoracic adenopathy or mild pulmonary infiltrates and stable lung function do not require treatment. Lofgren's syndrome typically requires supportive measures like rest, and NSAIDs or corticosteroids are specifically considered for persistent, debilitating arthritis.

SYSTEMIC CORTICOSTEROIDS

Systemic glucocorticoids are the first-line therapy for both pulmonary and extrapulmonary sarcoidosis. Their mechanism lies in suppressing macrophage and lymphocyte activity, dampening the production of cytokines like TNF-α and IFN-γ that participate in granulomatous inflammation.[5] Prednisone at 20 mg daily serves as the optimal starting dose, as no additional benefit has been demonstrated with higher dosages. In clinical practice, many centres worldwide initiate treatment with 20–40 mg prednisolone daily, with dose adjustments made for patients with comorbidities like diabetes, psychosis, or osteoporosis to mitigate potential side effects.[6] In sarcoidosis management, prednisone therapy should begin with a moderate dose, meticulously tapered to the lowest effective level, ideally below 10 mg daily. Maintaining this regimen for at least 6–24 months significantly reduces the risk of relapse associated with premature discontinuation.

The optimal tapering speed remains a subject of debate. While some advocate for slower approaches, recent evidence suggests that tapering the dose to 10 mg over 3.5 months offers similar efficacy and reduced steroid side effects.[7] Research by Broos et al further supports this, demonstrating a 7.4% improvement in forced vital capacity (FVC) within 3 months of starting prednisone therapy, regardless of the cumulative dose. Interestingly, this study also highlights a significant association between weight gain and higher cumulative doses, underscoring the importance of individualizing treatment plans.[8]

While moderate prednisone doses with meticulous tapering are optimal for sarcoidosis management, severe manifestations like neurosarcoidosis, vision-threatening eye disease, refractory arrhythmias, and other severe organ damage may require higher initial doses.[8] A Finnish study in pulmonary sarcoidosis used a protocol in which patients with Stage II–III disease received oral prednisolone for 3 months (20 mg daily for 8 weeks, 15 mg daily for 2 weeks, and 10 mg daily for 2 weeks) followed by inhaled budesonide for 15 months. This regimen demonstrated improved pulmonary function over five years, highlighting its potential benefits.[9] Higher cumulative doses of prednisone have been associated with decreased quality of life, increased emergency department visits, and even higher morbidity and mortality.[10,11] A study in Japan revealed increased morbidity and mortality in patients who were treated with higher doses of corticosteroids (>40 mg per day) compared to lower doses of corticosteroids (<30 mg per day).[11]

Steroid-sparing Medications

For patients intolerant to prednisone or experiencing therapeutic failure (inability to taper below 10 mg without worsening), recent ERS guidelines and Delphi consensus suggest transitioning to second-line therapies like methotrexate or other immunosuppressants like azathioprine (Fig. 6.1). A double-blind trial demonstrated that methotrexate does not worsen lung function but allows for reduced prednisone use and weight gain, highlighting its potential benefits.[12] If second-line agents are ineffective or poorly tolerated, third-line options like infliximab may be considered. Importantly, inhaled steroids offer no disease-modifying benefits but can improve cough and bronchial hyperreactivity in specific situations. Ultimately, steroid-sparing agents like methotrexate, azathioprine, or biologics become crucial for patients with steroid-refractory disease, relapse on tapering, or severe steroid side effects. This multi-tiered approach optimizes care by balancing disease control with minimizing long-term steroid risks.

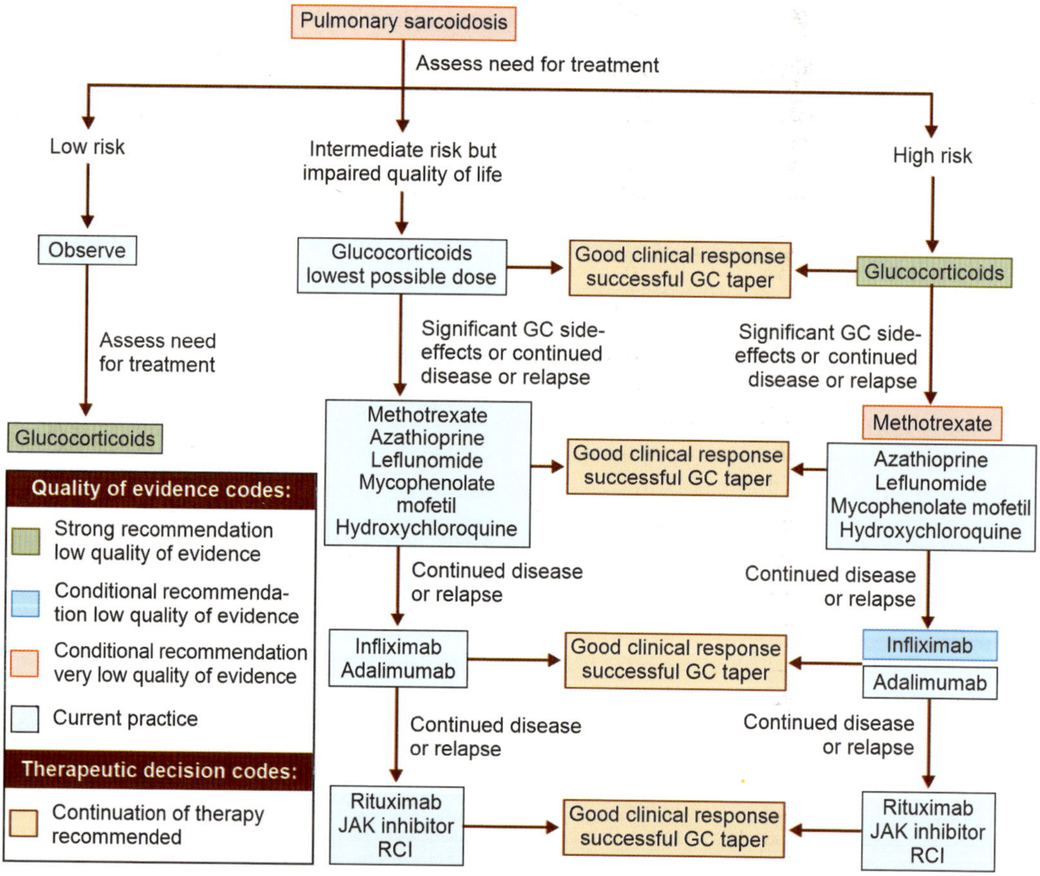

Fig. 6.1: The proposed algorithm for pulmonary sarcoidosis[3]

ACUTE PULMONARY EXACERBATIONS OF SARCOIDOSIS (APES)

Worsening respiratory symptoms in sarcoidosis patients are common, but accurately diagnosing acute pulmonary exacerbations of sarcoidosis (APES) requires careful differentiation. APES is a new or worsening granulomatous inflammation causing increased pulmonary symptoms accompanied by a >10% decline in FVC or FEV_1 compared to baseline (Panselinas and Judson's 2012 definition).[13] While "Acute" suggests symptoms lasting at least a month, and cough is present in >90% of patients, with fever and night sweats are rare.[14] Airway hyperreactivity may also be present in up to 58% of individuals. Diagnosing APES hinges on excluding alternative causes for symptom worsening. Ruling out extrapulmonary sarcoidosis involvement (e.g. cardiac or pulmonary hypertension), complications of immunosuppression, and other sarcoidosis-associated conditions like embolism, depression, fatigue, and small fiber neuropathy is crucial.

Corticosteroid therapy is the treatment of choice, although the exact dose and duration of therapy remain unknown. ERS, ATS, and WASOG guidelines recommend initial prednisone equivalents of 20–40 mg daily for pulmonary sarcoidosis. Studies suggest lower doses (e.g. 20 mg) may be effective for acute pulmonary exacerbations of sarcoidosis (APES) but carry less risk of long-term side effects like osteoporosis and cataracts. Corticosteroid-sparing agents should be considered in patients with multiple APES episodes (Fig. 6.2). A study by McKinzie et al showed rapid improvement in APES patients treated with prednisolone: Median time for normalizing pulmonary function was 21 days, with significant symptom improvement.[14] However, lack of response after 4–6 weeks necessitates exploring alternative diagnoses beyond APES.

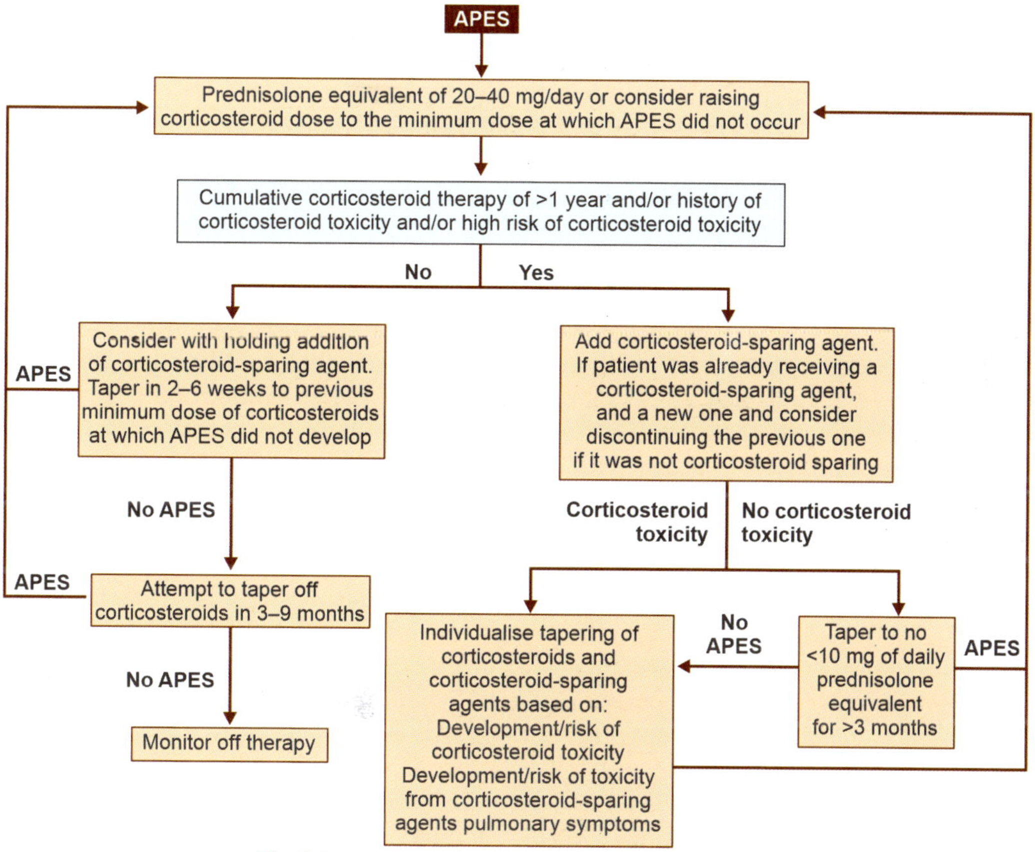

Fig. 6.2: A proposed treatment algorithm for APES[21]

Conclusion

Systemic corticosteroids are the mainstay of treatment for various sarcoidosis manifestations, including pulmonary, extrapulmonary, and life-threatening forms.

Evidence from randomized controlled trials supports their short-term effectiveness in improving lung function and chest X-ray findings in patients with progressive lung involvement. Alternative immunosuppressive agents (methotrexate or azathioprine) are considered for patients who do not respond adequately to corticosteroids.

HYPERSENSITIVITY PNEUMONITIS (HP)

Hypersensitivity pneumonitis (HP), also known as extrinsic allergic alveolitis, is an immune-mediated lung inflammation triggered by inhaling various organic or inorganic materials. It can lead to irreversible lung damage if left untreated. Recent guidelines from the ATS/JRS/ALAT and CHEST recommend classifying HP as fibrotic or non-fibrotic based on clinical, radiological, and pathological features.[15,16] The inflammatory response in HP involves both humoral and cellular mechanisms. Antigen exposure triggers innate immune processing, followed by a T-helper cell and antigen-specific IgG antibody-mediated response. This leads to lymphocyte accumulation and granuloma formation in the lungs.

Clinically, non-fibrotic HP features progressive dyspnea, fever, chills, chest tightness, wheezing, and weight loss over weeks to months. In contrast, fibrotic HP presents with a chronic cough and progressive exertional dyspnea developing over months to years. Both forms show a restrictive pattern on pulmonary function tests with impaired diffusing capacity for carbon monoxide (DLCO) and possibly some small airway obstruction in non-fibrotic cases.

There is no definitive pharmacological algorithm available for HP; corticosteroids remain the mainstay of initial HP treatment. While they may initially improve symptoms, evidence for long-term benefit or delaying progression, especially in fibrotic HP, is limited. Prednisone at a dose of 40–60 mg (0.5 mg/kg/day) daily, tapering until maintenance of 10 mg/day over 2–4 weeks, offers symptom relief and improved PFTs in non-fibrotic HP; its impact on fibrotic forms is negligible, highlighting the need for alternative approaches. A 2018 study by De Sadeleer et al supports this notion, demonstrating excellent outcomes in non-fibrotic patients with corticosteroid and antigen avoidance, while those with fibrotic disease showed minimal response.[17] Similarly, studies on farmers' lungs suggest short-term symptom relief with steroids and rapid radiological improvement but no long-term benefit.[18] Pharmacological treatment of fibrotic hypersensitivity pneumonitis (HP) presents significant challenges, despite the lack of strong evidence for any specific regimen. Corticosteroids, either alone or combined with azathioprine (AZA) or mycophenolate mofetil (MMF), remain the most frequently employed immunosuppressants in this setting. Importantly, combination therapy may offer a more favorable risk-benefit profile by reducing adverse events compared to monotherapy.[19] Notably, poor outcomes with corticosteroids were observed in fibrotic HP patients with low BAL lymphocytes and honeycombing on CT, highlighting the need for more personalized approaches.[20] Ultimately, the prognosis for fibrotic HP, like other fibrotic lung diseases, remains poor, emphasizing the importance of early diagnosis and antigen avoidance.

Conclusion

Current data suggests that corticosteroids are more beneficial for treating patients with predominantly non-fibrotic HP. However, they do not halt lung function decline and may be associated with increased mortality in patients with chronic fibrotic HP. Further research is crucial to optimize HP management across different disease stages and patient profiles. Importantly, antigen avoidance remains the cornerstone of HP management, regardless of corticosteroid response.

REFERENCES

1. Polverino F, Balestro E, Spagnolo P. Clinical Presentations, Pathogenesis, and Therapy of Sarcoidosis: State of the Art. J Clin Med. 2020 Jul 24;9(8):2363. doi: 10.3390/jcm9082363. PMID: 32722050; PMCID: PMC7465477.
2. American Thoracic Society, European Respiratory Society (ERS), and World Association of Sarcoidosis and Other Granulomatous Disorders. Statement on sarcoidosis. Joint Statement of the American Thoracic Society (ATS), the European Respiratory Society (ERS), and the World Association of Sarcoidosis and Other Granulomatous Disorders (WASOG) adopted by the ATS Board of Directors and by the ERS Executive Committee, February 1999. *Am J Respir Crit Care Med* 1999;160:736–755. doi: 10.1164/ajrccm.160.2.ats4-99.
3. Baughman RP, Valeyre D, Korsten P, et al. ERS clinical practice guidelines on treatment of sarcoidosis. *Eur Respir J* 2021;58:2004079.
4. Scadding JG. Prognosis of intrathoracic sarcoidosis in England. A review of 136 cases after five years' observation. *Br Med J* 1961;2:1165–72.
5. McKinzie BP, Bullington WM, Mazur JE, et al. Efficacy of short-course, low-dose corticosteroid therapy for acute pulmonary sarcoidosis exacerbations. *Am J Med Sci* 2010;339:1–4.
6. Rahaghi FF, Baughman RP, Saketkoo LA, et al. Delphi consensus recommendations for a treatment algorithm in pulmonary sarcoidosis. Eur Respir Rev 2020;29:190146.
7. Broos CE, Poell LHC, Looman CWN, et al. No evidence found for an association between prednisone dose and FVC change in newly-treated pulmonary sarcoidosis. Respir Med 2018;138S:S31–S37.
8. Schutt AC, Bullington WM, Judson MA. Pharmacotherapy for pulmonary sarcoidosis: a Delphi consensus study. Respir Med (2010) 104(5):717–23. doi: 10.1016/j.rmed.2009.12.009.
9. Pietinalho A, Tukiainen P, Haahtela T, Persson T, Selroos OFinnish Pulmonary Sarcoidosis Study G. Early treatment of stage II sarcoidosis improves 5-year pulmonary function. Chest (2002) 121(1): 24–31. doi: 10.1378/chest.121.1.24.
10. Judson MA, Chaudhry H, Louis A, Lee K, Yucel R. The effect of corticosteroids on quality of life in a sarcoidosis clinic: the results of a propensity analysis. Respir Med (2015) 109(4):526–31. doi: 10.1016/ j.rmed.2015.01.019.
11. Yazaki Y, Isobe M, Hiroe M, Morimoto S, Hiramitsu S, Nakano T, et al. Prognostic determinants of long-term survival in Japanese patients with cardiac sarcoidosis treated with prednisone. *Am J Cardiol* (2001) 88(9):1006–10. doi: 10.1016/S0002-9149(01)01978-6.
12. Baughman RP, Winget DB, Lower EE, Methotrexate is steroid sparing in acute sarcoidosis: results of a double blind, randomized trial, Sarcoidosis Vasc. Diffuse Lung Dis. 17(2000) 60–6.
13. Panselinas E, Judson MA. Acute pulmonary exacerbations of sarcoidosis. Chest 2012;142:827–836.
14. McKinzie BP, Bullington WM, Mazur JE, et al. Efficacy of short-course, low-dose corticosteroid therapy for acute pulmonary sarcoidosis exacerbations. *Am J Med Sci* 2010;339:1–4.
15. Raghu G, Remy-Jardin M, Ryerson CJ, et al. Diagnosis of hypersensitivity pneumonitis in adults. An official ATS/JRS/ALAT clinical practice guideline. Am J Respir Crit Care Med 2020; 202: e36–e69. doi:10.1164/rccm.202005-2032ST.
16. Fernández Pérez ER, Travis WD, Lynch DA, et al. Executive summary diagnosis and evaluation of hypersensitivity pneumonitis: CHEST guideline and expert panel report. Chest 2021; 160: 595–615. doi: 10.1016/j.chest.2021.03.067.
17. De Sadeleer L, Hermans F, De Dycker E, Yserbyt J, Verschakelen J, Verbeken E, et al. Effects of corticosteroid treatment and antigen avoidance in a large hypersensitivity pneumonitis cohort: a single-centre cohort study. *J Clin Med.* (2018) 8:14. doi: 10.3390/jcm8010014.

18. Mönkäre S, Haahtela T. Farmer's lung: a 5-year follow-up of eighty-six patients. Clin Allergy 1987; 17:143–151. doi:10.1111/j.1365-2222. 1987.tb02332.
19. Alberti ML, Rincon-Alvarez E, Buendia-Roldan I, Selman M. Hypersensitivity Pneumonitis: Diagnostic and Therapeutic Challenges. Front Med (Lausanne). 2021 Sep 23;8:718299. doi: 10.3389/fmed.2021.718299. PMID: 34631740; PMCID: PMC8495410.
20. De Sadeleer LJ, Hermans F, De Dycker E, et al. Impact of BAL lymphocytosis and presence of honeycombing on corticosteroid treatment effect in fibrotic hypersensitivity pneumonitis: a retrospective cohort study. *Eur Respir J* 2020;55:1901983. doi:10.1183/13993003.01983-2019.
21. Acute Pulmonary Exacerbations of Sarcoidosis. CHEST 2012;142(4):827–36.

Chapter 7

Steroids in Collagen Vascular Diseases

S Laxmi Kumari • Kakarla Bhaskar

INTRODUCTION

Connective tissue disorders are multisystemic immune-mediated disorders affecting joints, skin, serosal surfaces, renal, neurological systems, and lungs with variable manifestations and prognoses. Systemic lupus erythematosus (SLE), scleroderma, rheumatoid arthritis, mixed connective tissue disease (MCTD), Sjögren syndrome, and inflammatory myopathies (IIM) are the main disorders in this group. Pulmonary manifestations of these disorders involve all compartments, i.e. pleura, airways, alveoli, interstitium, pulmonary vessels, and respiratory muscles, including the diaphragm. The clinical course is further complicated by extrapulmonary involvement of other organs like kidneys, intervening infections due to immunosuppression, drug-induced lung disease, and malignancies.

RHEUMATOID ARTHRITIS INTERSTITIAL LUNG DISEASE (ILD)

Despite its primary manifestation as symmetric polyarthritis, rheumatoid arthritis (RA) extends beyond joint surfaces, with pleuropulmonary complications significantly impacting morbidity and mortality.[1] Interstitial lung disease (ILD) affects over 60% of RA patients, often remaining clinically silent initially.[2]

While HLA-DR susceptibility genes and smoking are strongly linked to anti-citrulline positive RA, specific genetic variants like MUC5B promoter polymorphism further increase susceptibility to RA-ILD development.[3] During inflammation, genetically predisposed individuals synthesize anti-citrullinated protein antibodies (ACPAs) found in most RA patients.[4] Serological markers like RA factor, anti-CCP, CRP, ESR, and KL-6 aid in diagnosis.

RA-ILD exhibits distinct radiological and histopathological phenotypes: a fibrotic disease with a UIP pattern and an inflammation-predominant disease with non-UIP patterns like NSIP and OP. Transbronchial cryobiopsies, with their high diagnostic yield and reduced risk, are emerging as a valuable tool for accurate diagnosis.[5]

Treatment

Management of RA includes steroids, conventional synthetic DMARDs (methotrexate, leflunomide, sulfasalazine, hydroxychloroquine), targeted synthetic DMARDs (tofacitinib, baricitinib, upadacitinib, filgotinib) and biologic DMARDs (TNF antagonists: Adalimumab, etanercept, golimumab, certolizumab, infliximab, IL-6 antagonists: Tocilizumab, Sarilumab, costimulation Inhibitor: Abatacept and CD20 antagonist: Rituximab). Consequently, treatment approaches require careful individualization. First-line therapy prioritizes symptom relief and inflammation control. Nonsteroidal anti-inflammatory drugs (NSAIDs) offer initial relief, but their impact on disease progression is limited. Corticosteroids, with their potent anti-inflammatory action, are more effective than NSAIDs but carry a higher risk of adverse effects. Their use is, therefore, cautious, often in short bursts or with careful tapering regimens. Second-line options, aiming for disease remission, focus on slowing or halting the progression of joint destruction and deformity.

Managing rheumatoid arthritis-interstitial lung disease (RA-ILD) presents a unique challenge due to the heterogeneous spectrum of clinical, radiological, and histological manifestations, coupled with the potential for iatrogenic exacerbation of symptoms. The therapeutic armamentarium for RA-ILD encompasses a diverse range of agents, including immunosuppressants, disease-modifying antirheumatic drugs (DMARDs), and biologicals. While the lack of robust evidence from randomized controlled trials (RCTs) presents a significant challenge, clinical experience and observational studies guide treatment selection. Corticosteroids, azathioprine, and mycophenolate mofetil remain the mainstay of therapy for RA-ILD patients due to their efficacy and relative tolerability. However, in refractory cases where conventional agents fail to achieve adequate disease control, rituximab or TNF-α inhibitors emerge as valuable alternatives, potentially offering superior efficacy through their targeted mechanisms of action.

The advent of highly efficacious DMARDs and biologicals has reshaped the therapeutic landscape for RA-ILD, shifting the primary objective from mere inflammation control to achieving disease remission.[6,7] Early initiation of combination therapy involving corticosteroids alongside DMARDs or biologicals demonstrates superior efficacy compared to DMARD monotherapy. Studies have shown this approach to not only induce higher remission rates but also control radiological progression more effectively.[8]

The 2008 British Thoracic Society (BTS) guidelines advocate for prednisone as the first-line treatment for RA-ILD, with a starting dose of 0.5 mg/kg/day for 1–3 months, followed by careful tapering to 10 mg/day or less in combination with DMARDs (Fig. 7.1). This approach prioritizes initial inflammation control while minimizing steroid-related adverse effects.[9] In cases of corticosteroid failure, the guidelines recommend adding an immunosuppressant agent like cyclosporine, azathioprine, or cyclophosphamide to enhance therapeutic efficacy. Notably, higher-dose steroids may be considered for rapidly progressing inflammatory subtypes of RA-ILD, such as cellular NSIP and organizing pneumonia, during their acute or subacute presentations.

In rheumatoid arthritis-associated interstitial lung disease (RA-ILD), corticosteroids remain the mainstay of therapy, administered either daily or in pulsed courses tapered over months based on individual tolerance and response. Other immunosuppressants like TNF-α inhibitors, methotrexate, azathioprine, mycophenolate mofetil, and cyclophosphamide are reserved for maintenance therapy or steroid-resistant cases.[10] While limited data exists from retrospective case series, the combination of methylprednisolone and cyclophosphamide might offer potential benefits for severe

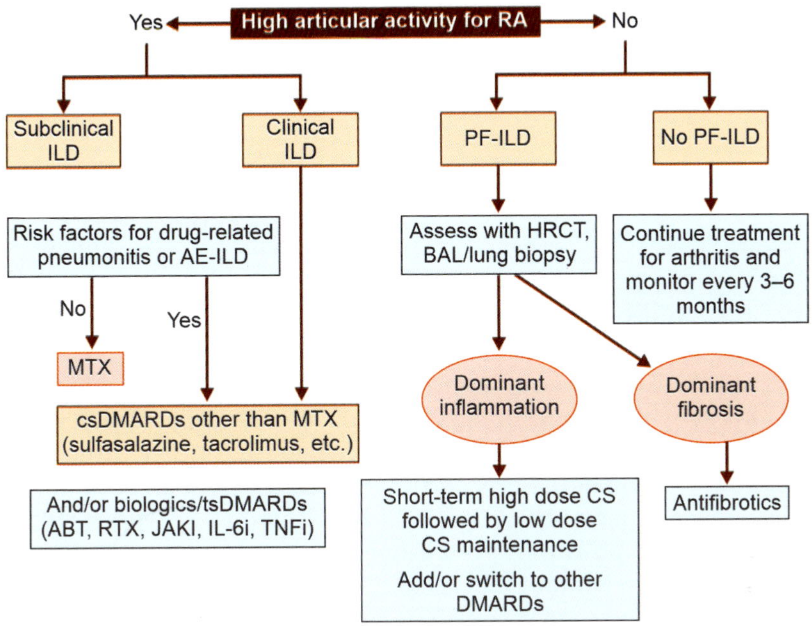

Fig. 7.1: Decision-making strategy for treatment of chronic RA-ILD

MTX: Methotrexate; **ABT:** Abatacept; **RTX:** Rituximab; **csDMARs:** Conventional synthetic DMARDs; **tsDMARDs:** Targeted synthetic DMARDs; **CS:** Corticosteroids; **JAKi:** Janus kinase inhibitors; **IL-6i:** Interleukin-6 inhibitors; **TNFi:** Tumor necrosis factor inhibitors.

RA-ILD with extensive UIP and rapid progression.[11] Additionally, intra-articular steroid injections remain a valuable option for managing localized inflammation.[12]

A meta-analysis by Finckh et al demonstrated a significant 33% reduction in radiographic progression among patients who received DMARDs within the first two years of disease onset compared to those treated later.[13] These benefits persisted for up to five years, highlighting the crucial window for early intervention. Svensson et al study investigated the impact of adding low-dose prednisolone (7.5 mg daily) to DMARD therapy at treatment initiation for patients with active RA and a disease duration of ≤1 year. After 2 years, radiographic progression was significantly lower in the prednisolone group (25.9% vs 39.3%). Additionally, remission rates were considerably higher (55.5% vs. 32.8%).[14] Harfstrom et al study similar to Svensson et al this study found a significantly higher remission rate at 2 years in the prednisolone group compared to the control group (55% vs. 30%). Notably, bone density changes did not differ significantly between the groups over 4 years.[15] A systematic review further supports the benefits of glucocorticoid incorporation along with standard therapy, demonstrating a significant reduction in the incidence of progressive erosions in RA patients treated with this combined approach.[16]

RA Pleurisy and Pleural Effusion

Pleural effusions may manifest unilaterally or bilaterally, often concomitant with the presence of interstitial lung disease. These effusions typically present as exudates, characterized by a low pleural fluid pH and glucose concentration.

There are no control studies evaluating the efficacy of steroids or NSAIDs in the treatment of RA pleural effusion. In only symptomatic patients, the treatment should be therapeutic thoracocentesis and intrapleural corticosteroids. Nevertheless, it is noteworthy that corticosteroids, employed as part of the therapeutic regimen for active articular disease, concurrently demonstrate efficacy in expediting the resolution of pleural effusions.

Pulmonary Vascular Disease

Pleuropulmonary complications associated with rheumatoid arthritis and pulmonary vascular disease stand out as a relatively rare occurrence. However, when it does manifest, it is often accompanied by the presence of Raynaud phenomenon.

The recommended therapeutic approach involves the initial administration of intravenous methylprednisolone, followed by oral corticosteroid preparations. Additionally, the incorporation of cyclophosphamide into the treatment regimen is deemed necessary for managing this particular complication. In accordance with the observations made in other systemic vasculitides, rituximab can induce remission and concomitantly reduce exposure to prednisone in a significant proportion of patients grappling with systemic rheumatoid vasculitis.[17]

Airway Involvement in RA

RA involves airways starting from the upper airway by involving the cricoarytenoid joint. Bronchiolitis obliterans (BO) is a recognized contributor to severe progressive obstructive airway disease among individuals with RA.[18] It is the initial manifestation in a few patients and has more predilection in females.[19] It is treated with steroids and cyclophosphamide and has a poor prognosis as it may lead to hypercapnic respiratory failure. Follicular bronchiolitis and diffuse pan bronchiolitis are also observed and are treated with steroids.

SYSTEMIC LUPUS ERYTHEMATOSUS

Systemic lupus erythematosus (SLE), an autoimmune disease characterized by self-targeting antibodies and immune complexes, can involve the lungs in various ways, with interstitial lung disease (ILD) being a less common but potentially severe manifestation. Other pulmonary presentations in SLE include pleuritis, thromboembolism, alveolar hemorrhage, and, on a less frequent basis, shrinking lung syndrome. Diagnosis relies on the 2019 EULAR/ACR criteria, combining clinical features and serological findings.

Pathogenesis

While the exact mechanisms underlying lung involvement in SLE remain unclear, distinct features emerge. ILD in SLE is associated with aberrant remodelling of lung tissue due to excessive extracellular matrix deposition and impaired epithelial cell repair after injury. Additionally, elevated levels of proinflammatory cytokines like IFN-γ, TNF-α, IL-6, IL-8, and IL-12 contribute to the inflammatory milieu.[20] Interestingly, research suggests that specific extractable nuclear antigens (ENA), namely anti-La, anti-Scl-70, and anti-U1RNP, might be associated with an increased risk of ILD development, while anti-dsDNA antibody levels do not seem to be predictive.[21]

Treatment

Due to the absence of established guidelines, recommendations for SLE-ILD therapy primarily rely on case reports, small series, expert opinions, and studies on ILD in other autoimmune rheumatic diseases. The European League Against Rheumatism (EULAR) advocates hydroxychloroquine as first-line therapy for all SLE patients, with glucocorticoids added as needed.[22] Immunosuppressants are reserved for refractory cases or life-threatening situations as initial therapy.

In severe cases of SLE-ILD, a short burst of high-dose corticosteroids, known as pulse therapy, can be crucial to dampen the inflammatory storm. This typically involves either prednisolone at 0.5–1 mg/kg/day or intravenous methylprednisolone at 0.5–1 g daily for 3 days. Following pulse therapy, the goal is to taper down the steroid dosage to the minimum effective dose (usually 7.5–5 mg/day) while simultaneously initiating steroid-sparing agents to maintain disease control and minimize steroid-related side effects. Some commonly used steroid-sparing agents in SLE-ILD include MMF, azathioprine, belimumab, rituximab, and tacrolimus.

Corticosteroids should be considered as first-line therapy along with cyclophosphamide (CYC) or mycophenolate mofetil (MMF), followed by either rituximab or intravenous immunoglobulin (IVIg).[23,24] In mild and moderate SLE-ILD, Koo et al advocate for first-line therapy with corticosteroids, transitioning to azathioprine or MMF for maintenance. In refractory cases, high-dose corticosteroids combined with steroid-sparing agents, primarily cyclophosphamide, may be necessary.[25,26] Weinrib et al demonstrated improved vital capacity and DLCO in some patients treated with high-dose oral prednisolone despite limited overall evidence of efficacy.[27] While its effectiveness remains debated, corticosteroids are frequently employed empirically alongside immunosuppressants in clinical trials.

SJÖGREN'S SYNDROME

Sjögren's syndrome (SS) is characterized by autoimmune inflammation of epithelial tissues and heightened B cell activity, resulting in reduced function of exocrine glands. Pulmonary manifestations in Sjögren's syndrome include dry airway mucosa leading to bronchitis sicca, increased lymphocytic activity leading to follicular bronchiolitis, LIP, and an increased risk of lymphoma. Nonspecific interstitial pneumonia (NSIP) is the most common radiological finding.

Treatment

Steroids remain the cornerstone of therapy for Sjögren's syndrome-ILD, serving as first-line treatment in most cases. The initial dose typically ranges from 0.5 to 1 mg/kg/day, adjusted based on disease severity.[28] This approach balances effectiveness in controlling inflammation with minimizing steroid-related side effects. To minimize steroid-related side effects and potentially improve response, corticosteroids may be combined with immunosuppressants like azathioprine or others.[28] Rituximab may be considered in patients with refractory disease or those unresponsive to initial therapy.[29] Interestingly, the response to treatment varies based on the underlying ILD pattern. Patients with NSIP, organizing pneumonia (OP), and lymphocytic interstitial pneumonia (LIP) patterns generally exhibit better responses to immunosuppressive therapy, including steroids, compared to those with usual interstitial pneumonia (UIP) patterns.

SYSTEMIC SCLEROSIS

Systemic sclerosis, also known as scleroderma, is an autoimmune disease characterized by inflammation and excessive deposition of extracellular matrix (ECM) in various organs. This leads to fibrosis, or hardening, of the skin and internal tissues. The disease can affect the lungs, heart, kidneys, gastrointestinal tract, and more. There are two main forms of scleroderma: diffuse cutaneous scleroderma, which involves widespread skin thickening, and limited cutaneous scleroderma, which primarily affects the hands and face.[30] Understanding the specific type and extent of organ involvement is crucial for guiding treatment and managing the diverse complications associated with this complex disease.

Pathophysiology

While the exact mechanisms behind systemic sclerosis (SSc) remain under investigation, the interplay between immune cells, endothelial cells, and fibroblasts plays a key role.[31] The hallmark feature, seen both in the lungs and skin, is an abnormal accumulation of connective tissue cells and proteins. This surge is mainly driven by the upregulation of TGF-β, a potent stimulator of collagen production, particularly evident in the lungs of SSc patients. Additionally, elevated levels of endothelin-1 (ET-1), proteins associated with coagulation, and proinflammatory cytokines like IL-8, TNF-α, and MIP-1α are found in bronchoalveolar lavage fluid.[32]

Radiologically, the most common finding is the nonspecific interstitial pneumonia (NSIP) pattern, followed by usual interstitial pneumonia (UIP). Patients with extensive disease are at higher risk of mortality and lung function decline. Interestingly, almost all individuals with SSc-ILD have positive antinuclear antibodies, often accompanied by specific autoantibodies like anti-Scl-70, anti-Th/To, anti-U3 RNP, anti-U11/U12 RNP, and rarely anti-centromere antibodies. This complex interplay between signaling pathways, inflammatory mediators, and autoantibodies highlights the need for further research to unravel the pathogenesis of SSc and develop targeted therapies.

Treatment

Given the understanding that inflammation precedes and drives fibrosis in SSc-ILD, with only the inflammatory component considered reversible, early treatment is paramount. However, fibrosis often dominates the clinical picture.

The scleroderma lung study demonstrated modest but significant improvement in FVC, skin scores, quality of life, and dyspnea with oral cyclophosphamide (2 mg/kg/day, max 150 mg) compared to placebo at 12 months, often combined with low-dose prednisolone (10 mg/day or 20 mg every other day).[33,34] Intravenous cyclophosphamide (750–1000 mg/m^2) every 2–4 weeks for 6–12 months may offer a better safety profile. The Scleroderma Lung Study II showed comparable efficacy between MMF and cyclophosphamide over 1–2 years, with MMF being better tolerated and therefore preferred as first-line therapy by many.[35] A single-centre study found a 158 ml average improvement in FVC for patients receiving continuous corticosteroids over 1 year compared to a 61 ml decline in those who did not. However, long-term use (>10 mg/day) carries a significant risk of scleroderma renal crisis.[36]

The use of corticosteroids in SSc-ILD remains a complex and controversial issue. While their potential benefits for symptom control and lung function improvement are undeniable, concerns regarding side effects and, particularly, scleroderma renal crisis (SRC) necessitate careful consideration. Observational data from EUSTAR (European Scleroderma Trials and Research Group) suggests that over half of SSc-ILD patients receive steroid doses exceeding 20 mg/day, with modest improvements in FVC, especially for those with FVC >75%. However, long-term use of even 10 mg/day prednisolone carries a significant risk of scleroderma renal crisis.[37,38]

The controversy primarily surrounds the use of corticosteroids in early diffuse SSc (dcSSc). This subgroup may benefit most from symptom relief, as itching and musculoskeletal issues often respond well, but also faces the highest scleroderma renal crisis risk. The PRedSS study (PRednisolone in early diffuse systemic sclerosis), while inconclusive, suggests short-term moderate-dose prednisolone for symptom control in early dcSSc may be considered, highlighting the need for further research to optimize steroid use in this vulnerable population.[39]

INFLAMMATORY MYOPATHIES

Idiopathic inflammatory myopathies (IIMs), a diverse group encompassing polymyositis (PM), dermatomyositis (DM), anti-synthetase syndrome, immune-mediated necrotizing myopathy (IMIN), and inclusion body myositis, are rare autoimmune conditions characterized by skeletal muscle inflammation.[40] Interestingly, the most common pulmonary complication associated with IIMs, occurring in roughly 45% of patients and representing the leading cause of death, is interstitial lung disease (ILD).

Histopathological analysis of ILD in IIM patients reveals a diverse range of patterns. Nonspecific interstitial pneumonia (NSIP) is the most prevalent pattern, observed in a staggering 82% of cases. Other less common patterns include usual interstitial pneumonia (UIP) in patients with extensive fibrosis, diffuse alveolar damage in acute pneumonitis, and organizing pneumonia. Understanding these distinct histopathological presentations is crucial for accurate diagnosis and optimal management of IIM-associated ILD, ultimately improving patient outcomes.

Treatment

Treatment for interstitial lung disease (ILD) associated with idiopathic inflammatory myopathies (IIMs) depends heavily on the underlying histology. Cellular disease, characterized by increased inflammatory cell infiltration, generally responds better to therapy.[41] Corticosteroids, potent anti-inflammatory drugs, are the cornerstone of initial treatment due to their rapid onset of action and manageable side effects. A study by Lundberg et al reported that oral prednisolone (0.25–1 mg/kg) for 3–8 weeks, followed by a gradual taper, led to clinical improvement in 90–100% of patients with cellular ILD.[42]

For mild cases with progressive disease or moderate ILD, prednisolone 1 mg/kg daily is often combined with mycophenolate mofetil (MMF) or azathioprine, with steroid duration typically lasting 4–6 months.[43] While monotherapy with corticosteroids has a reported response rate of 37.5–52%, with polymyositis patients generally responding better than dermatomyositis patients, it alone may not be sufficient for all cases.[44] A systematic review and meta-analysis found that steroids yielded functional improvement in 89% of patients, but their use in rapidly progressive ILD (RP-ILD) was associated with lower survival rates compared to other immunosuppressive agents.[40,41] Therefore, for patients who do not respond well to steroids alone or whose disease persists, alternative options like tacrolimus and rituximab are considered.

For patients with ILD progressing to severe hypoxemia and respiratory failure, aggressive therapy with multiple agents is necessary. This may involve pulse dose methylprednisolone followed by 1 mg/kg prednisolone daily, along with intravenous immunoglobulins (IVIg) at 2 g/kg in divided doses and an additional steroid-sparing agent.[43,45] High-dose steroids should be maintained for 2–4 weeks and then gradually reduced until reaching a maintenance dose of 5–10 mg/day prednisolone.[45]

In rapidly progressive ILD (RP-ILD) associated with IIMs, rituximab emerges as the first-line therapy due to its efficacy.[46] Other immunosuppressants like cyclophosphamide, cyclosporine, and tacrolimus have also shown promise for steroid-resistant cases. Notably, Kurita et al found tacrolimus associated with superior long-term progression-free and event-free survival compared to steroid monotherapy or combinations with other immunosuppressants.[47] In refractory cases, methotrexate and intravenous immunoglobulins may be considered.[44]

ANTI-SYNTHETASE SYNDROME (ASSD)

Anti-synthetase syndrome (ASSD) exhibits a high prevalence of ILD, with specific autoantibodies like PL-7 and PL-12 often linked to greater severity. Compared to other ILDs associated with idiopathic inflammatory myositis (IIM), ASSD-ILD shows both enhanced treatment response and a higher risk of recurrence.[48] Notably, Jo-1, PL-7, PL-12, EJ, and OJ antibodies all demonstrate an association with ILD presence.

In an Italian study, Jo-1-positive patients with ILD received cyclosporine after failing steroid monotherapy. After one year, they experienced improvements in DLCO, FVC, and HRCT scores. Ingegnoli et al study compared two treatment regimens for 15 patients with Jo-1-positive ILD. Seven received steroids + cyclosporine, while eight received steroids and intravenous cyclophosphamide. Interestingly, HRCT worsened in half of the CYC group and 71% of the cyclosporine group.[49] Chen et al study presented a different perspective, with 3 out of 5 subjects responding positively to steroids and the cyclophosphamide combination.[50]

Recent work by Hozumi et al utilized propensity score analysis to compare initial treatment strategies in ASSD (adult-onset Still's disease) patients with ILD. They found that a combination of glucocorticoids and calcineurin inhibitors led to significantly improved progression-free survival compared to steroids alone, although no significant difference in long-term survival was observed.[51]

MIXED CONNECTIVE TISSUE DISEASE (MCTD)

Mixed connective tissue disease (MCTD) presents a diagnostic and therapeutic challenge due to its overlapping features with systemic sclerosis (SSc), systemic lupus erythematosus (SLE), rheumatoid arthritis (RA), and polymyositis/dermatomyositis (PM/DM). Notably, anti-ribonucleoprotein (RNP) antibodies are a hallmark of MCTD and play a potential role in its pathogenesis.

Interstitial lung disease (ILD) is a frequent and potentially life-threatening complication in MCTD, affecting up to 80% of patients. While definitive data regarding

MCTD-ILD treatment remains limited, immunosuppressive therapy, similar to other connective tissue diseases (CTDs), plays a crucial role. Immunosuppressive therapy plays a central role in managing MTCD-ILD, with corticosteroids and steroid-sparing agents being the mainstays. Corticosteroids often serve as first-line therapy due to their rapid response and efficacy in controlling inflammation. Starting doses around 0.5 mg/kg/day prednisolone are typical, with subsequent tapering based on individual response and disease severity. To minimize long-term steroid exposure and its associated adverse effects, steroid-sparing agents like cyclophosphamide (CYC) and azathioprine (AZA) are often combined with corticosteroids.[52] The choice and dosage of steroid-sparing agents are individualized based on disease severity, response to corticosteroids, and patient tolerability.

ANCA-ASSOCIATED VASCULITIDES (AAV)

ANCA-associated vasculitides include granulomatosis with polyangiitis (GPA), microscopic polyangiitis (MPA), and eosinophilic granulomatosis with polyangiitis (EGPA).

1. Granulomatosis with Polyangiitis/Microscopic Polyangiitis (GPA/MPA)

Among ANCA-associated vasculitides, GPA reigns as the most common lung vasculitis. This autoimmune disorder is characterized by necrotizing granulomatous inflammation, typically involving the respiratory tract, and necrotizing vasculitis, predominantly affecting small to medium vessels. Upper airways (90–95%), lungs (54–85%), and kidneys (51–80%) are frequently involved, though any organ can be affected. While previously categorized as "non-severe" and "severe," current terminology distinguishes between presentations with or without organ-threatening or life-threatening diseases (Fig. 7.2).[53] In "non-severe" GPA, biopsies primarily show necrotizing granulomatous inflammation with less clinical significance, while "severe" GPA presents a life-threatening or irreversible damage risk to vital organs.

In contrast, microscopic polyangiitis (MPA) can affect any organ but primarily targets the kidneys (80%). Diffuse alveolar hemorrhage (DAH) occurs in 10–30% of patients, making MPA the most frequent cause of pulmonary-renal syndrome.

Pathophysiology

The development of ANCA-associated vasculitis involves a complex interplay of factors. Genetic predisposition to autoimmunity, epigenetic influences, and environmental triggers all contribute to the disease process. Infections or other environmental exposures can trigger a loss of self-tolerance, leading to an inflammatory environment that, in susceptible individuals, drives the production of autoantibodies known as antineutrophil cytoplasmic antibodies (ANCAs).[54]

Diagnosing active disease relies on a combination of clinical symptoms, chest CT findings, ANCA presence (cANCA or pANCA), and biopsy specimens from affected organs. Notably, MPA exhibits a higher prevalence of ILD compared to GPA, highlighting the importance of accurate diagnosis for guiding optimal treatment strategies.[55]

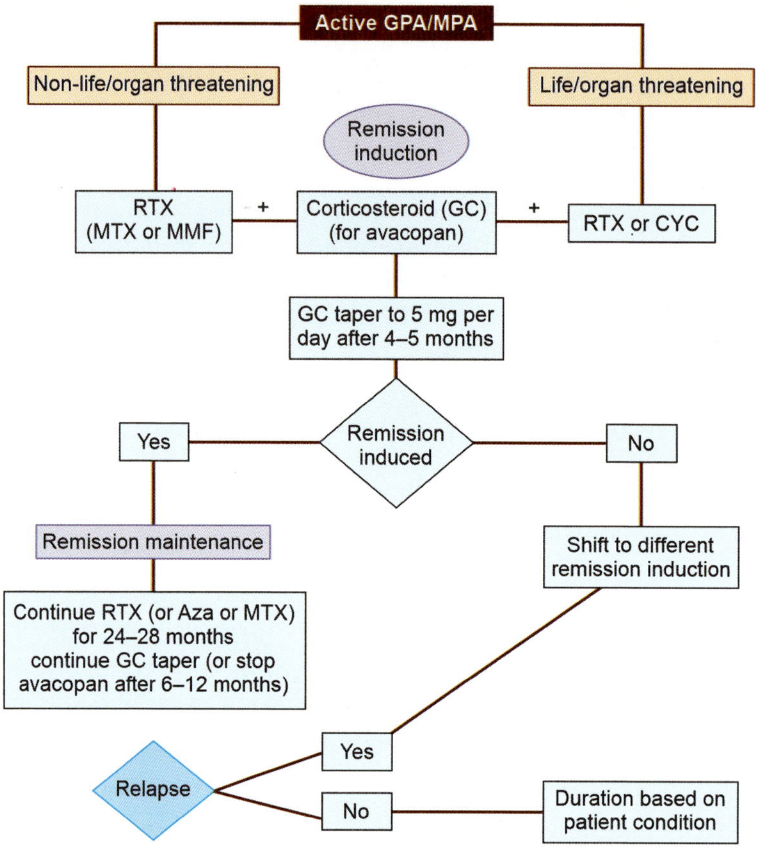

Fig. 7.2: Treatment algorithm for GPA/MPA (2022 EULAR)

RTX: Rituximab; **CYC:** cyclophosphamide; **MTX:** Methotrexate; **MMF:** Mycophenolate mofetil; **Aza:** Azathioprine

Treatment

Steroids are the mainstay of treatment in GPA/MPA.

Induction of Remission

Non-life-threatening GPA/MPA: For non-life-threatening granulomatosis with polyangiitis (GPA) and microscopic polyangiitis (MPA), treatment aims at achieving remission with minimal side effects and maximizing long-term disease control. A multipronged approach often includes glucocorticoids, immunosuppressants, and emerging agents like C5a complement inhibitors.

Prednisolone is the mainstay therapy that starts at 1 mg/kg/day (50~75 mg/day) or an equivalent dosage of other steroids. A stepwise reduction follows, aiming to reach 5 mg daily within 4–5 months.[56] The PEXIVAS study outlines specific dosing based on body weight and treatment week (Table 7.1).

While rituximab offers the advantage of higher sustained remission rates and lower steroid dependence compared to methotrexate or mycophenolate mofetil, the NORAM trial established methotrexate as a non-inferior alternative for induction.[57,58] However, methotrexate carries a higher risk of relapse.[59]

Table 7.1: Prednisolone mg/day tapering in GPA/MPA (PEXIVAS)			
Weeks	*Body weight (kg)*		
	<50 kg	50–75 kg	>75 kg
1	50 mg/day	60 mg/day	75 mg/day
2	25	30	40
3–4	20	25	30
5–6	15	20	25
7–8	12.5	15	20
9–10	10	12.5	15
11–12	7.5	10	12.5
13–14	6	7.5	10
15–18	5	5	7.5
19–52	5	5	5
>52	Individual taper	Individual taper	Individual taper

C5aR inhibitor avacopan: Emerging evidence suggests that the C5a inhibitor avacopan, administered at 30 mg twice daily alongside rituximab or cyclophosphamide, may offer a steroid-sparing approach in non-life-threatening GPA/MPA. Studies indicate that combining avacopan with a 1 mg/kg/day prednisolone regimen tapered over 21 weeks leads to fewer side effects, better kidney function recovery, and a higher rate of sustained remission at 52 weeks compared to standard steroid-only regimens.[60] Notably, avacopan appears to demonstrate superior efficacy in maintaining remission, although further research is needed to assess its long-term safety beyond 1 year. Additionally, ADVOCATE and CLEAR trials establish its non-inferiority to steroids, highlighting its potential as a potential steroid-sparing option.[61–63]

CYCAZAREM trial suggests oral cyclophosphamide with glucocorticoids for 3–6 months achieves similar relapse rates as 12 months of azathioprine, though relapses are more frequent in GPA compared to MPA.[64] Plasma exchange may be necessary for patients with severe manifestations like serum creatinine exceeding 300 µmol/L. Plasma exchange is also recommended for AAV patients with positive anti-GBM autoantibodies.[65]

Life-threatening GPA/MPA

In life-threatening GPA/MPA, rapid remission within 3 months is crucial for optimal outcomes. Delayed remission, early relapse, or refractory disease pose significant risks. Treatment strategies prioritize potent immunosuppression while minimizing long-term toxicity.[66]

According to the PEXIVAS trial, pulsed methylprednisolone therapy (1000–3000 mg daily for 3–5 days) to severe manifestations, particularly active renal involvement with eGFR <50 ml/min/1.73 m^2 or diffuse alveolar hemorrhage (DAH). While a 3-day pulse followed by oral glucocorticoids remains common practice, the initial dose for severe disease is now 1 mg/kg daily prednisone (or equivalent). Importantly, the PEXIVAS trial demonstrated that rapid dose reduction to 20 mg daily by 7 weeks and 5 mg daily by 19 weeks is equally effective and safer than traditional high-dose regimens.[67]

The combination of cyclophosphamide and glucocorticoids remains a mainstay for inducing remission in ANCA-associated vasculitis, typically achieving success within 3–6 months. Maintenance therapy for 12–36 months after remission, with longer durations, is recommended for high-risk relapse patients. Glucocorticoids plus Rituximab or cyclophosphamide are useful in relapsing cases.[68]

The RAVE trial established rituximab as a viable alternative for remission induction, with a recommended dosage of 375 mg/m^2 intravenously administered weekly for four weeks (weeks 0, 1, 2, 3). Growing concerns about the long-term safety of cyclophosphamide further favour the use of rituximab in many cases. Limited data on cyclophosphamide vs rituximab in low GFR (<20 ml/min/1.73 m^2) patients. RITUXVAS trial suggests using a lower cyclophosphamide dose alongside rituximab in these cases.[69]

Maintenance of Remission

Maintaining remission in life-threatening GPA/MPA involves continued immunosuppression after induction therapy, tailored to individual needs and relapse patterns.

Rituximab or cyclophosphamide for 24–48 months following induction, along with low-dose steroids. According to the MAINRITSAN trail, the recommended dosage of rituximab for remission maintenance is 500 mg every 6 months for 18 to 36 months.[70–72] Longer duration of treatment is considered in relapsing patients. Azathioprine or methotrexate are other alternatives.

For relapsing cases: In cases of relapsing ANCA-associated vasculitis, the RITAZAREM trial brought promising news. Glucocorticoids paired with rituximab showed efficacy, even for severe presentations, with lower initial steroid doses (0.5 mg/kg daily) and maintenance rituximab (1,000 mg every 4 months for 2 years), offering a potentially safer approach.[73,74]

For refractory cases: Refractory disease is defined as a failure to achieve full control of vasculitis-related disease activity by 6 months, progression of disease within first 3 months, or relapse despite adequate ongoing maintenance therapy.[75]

ILD with positive ANCA but not meeting MPA criteria: These patients often receive individualized therapy with low-dose corticosteroids alone or combined with various agents like azathioprine, cyclosporine, colchicine, infliximab, or interferon-γ, mizoribine or N-acetylcysteine.[76–78] The main indication for immunosuppression is progressive respiratory failure.

In severe relapse, high-dose intravenous glucocorticoids like methylprednisolone can be used for initial control, but prolonged high-dose oral corticosteroids should be avoided due to their side effects. Consider switching between cyclophosphamide and rituximab based on individual response and tolerability. PEXIVAS study discourages routine plasma exchange for GPA or MPA with nephritis or lung hemorrhage; specific subgroups like oliguric patients or those with hypoxic respiratory failure may benefit, and further research is warranted for refractory ANCA-associated vasculitis (AAV) in a study where high-dose intravenous immunoglobulin (IVIg) therapy (2 g/kg total dose) showed promise in improving disease control. Emerging evidence suggests a potential role for high-dose IVIg (2 g/kg total dose) in improving disease control in refractory cases.[79]

2. Eosinophilic Granulomatosis with Polyangiitis (EGPA)

Introduction

Eosinophilic granulomatosis with polyangiitis (EGPA), previously known by various terms like Churg-Strauss syndrome, presents a diverse clinical picture with historical terms like "allergic granulomatosis" and "allergic angiitis," reflecting its multifaceted nature. Characterized by blood and tissue eosinophilia, granulomatous inflammation, and allergic sensitization, EGPA triggers vasculitis and necrosis, often affecting the lungs.[80] Notably, EGPA's high prevalence of asthma and peripheral/tissue eosinophilia distinguishes it from GPA and MPA. Interestingly, the disease follows a three-phase course (asthma, eosinophilic, systemic vasculitis) but not always sequentially, adding to its complexity.

Pathophysiology

The pathogenesis of EGPA remains multifaceted, involving both autoimmune processes and environmental influences. In ANCA-positive EGPA, a Th2-mediated inflammatory response takes centre stage, potentially driven by genetic susceptibility linked to MHC DRB4, DRB1*04, and DRB1*07 alleles.[81,82] However, even in ANCA-negative cases, genetic variations impacting IL-10 expression, Th17 dysregulation, clonal expansion of CD8+/Vβ+ T cells, and specific T cell abnormalities suggest a complex interplay beyond ANCA presence.[83–85] Beyond genetics, environmental triggers play a significant role. Vaccines, allergens, infections (aspergillosis, ascariasis), and exposure to silica, birds, or smoked cocaine have all been linked to EGPA development. Additionally, drug-induced EGPA has been reported with medications like macrolides, sulphonamides, propylthiouracil, immune checkpoint inhibitors, and even leukotriene receptor antagonists.[86–88]

Treatment

In eosinophilic granulomatosis with polyangiitis (EGPA), treatment is guided by the severity of the disease. The French Vasculitis Study Group's Five-Factor Score (FFS) serves as a valuable prognostic tool, guiding therapeutic decisions.[89] Each present factor (renal insufficiency, significant gastrointestinal involvement, cardiac symptoms, lack of upper airway involvement, age >65) adds one point to the score, offering a comprehensive assessment of disease severity. Management strategies then diverge based on FFS and disease manifestations.

Remission Induction and Maintenance of Non-Life-threatening Manifestations

In EGPA patients with a favorable prognosis (FFS = 0), initial remission induction can be achieved with low-dose glucocorticoid monotherapy. This starts with prednisolone at 1 mg/kg/day for 3 weeks (maximum 80 mg/day), followed by a gradual tapering schedule: 7.5 mg reduction every two weeks until reaching 0.25 mg/kg/day after 3 months, then 5 mg reduction every 2 weeks until 10 mg/day, and finally 1 mg reduction every 3 weeks to the lowest effective dose. This strategy has demonstrated remarkable efficacy, with remission rates exceeding 93% in clinical trials.[90,91]

For EGPA patients with higher disease severity (FFS ≥1), the REOVAS study demonstrated that rituximab (1000 mg pulses every two weeks) achieved comparable remission rates to cyclophosphamide (nine intravenous pulses over five months) when combined with low-dose prednisone (≤7.5 mg daily). Notably, both ANCA-positive and ANCA-negative patients responded favorably to rituximab, offering a potential alternative to cyclophosphamide in this patient group.[92]

Additional immunosuppressive therapy is needed in severe disease only. If the FFS score is >2 or if refractory disease or disease that flares with steroid tapers, add cyclophosphamide to improve survival.

Remission Induction of Life-threatening Manifestations

For EGPA patients facing potentially fatal complications, rapid and intensive treatment is essential to prevent further damage and achieve remission. The standard approach typically involves a combination of high-dose corticosteroids and either cyclophosphamide (600 mg/m^2 administered on days 1, 15, and 29, followed by 500 mg every 15–20 days) or rituximab (1 g administered on days 1 and 15).[92]

Randomized controlled trials in patients with FFS ≥1 have suggested optimizing cyclophosphamide dosing for improved relapse-free survival. Research indicates that 12 pulses of cyclophosphamide (administered every 2 weeks for 1 month, then every 4 weeks thereafter, at a dose of 0.6 g/m^2 per pulse) offer a longer remission duration compared to 6 pulses.[93] Remission is typically achieved within 6 months of initiating therapy.

Furthermore, the French Vasculitis Study Group suggests that, in patients with higher FFS scores, employing cyclophosphamide for remission induction demonstrably improves overall survival.[94,95]

Maintenance of Remission of Life-threatening Manifestations

Following remission induction for life-threatening EGPA manifestations, various maintenance strategies can be employed to prevent disease flare-ups. Methotrexate (15–20 mg weekly orally/subcutaneously), azathioprine (2 mg/kg/day), or newer agents like mepolizumab, rituximab, or leflunomide offer options with varying immunosuppressive profiles.[96] However, rituximab necessitates monitoring serum immunoglobulins before each dose to detect potential secondary immunodeficiency.[97]

All AAV patients who receive cyclophosphamide, rituximab, or prednisolone >30 mg/day for >4 weeks need to take prophylaxis with trimethoprim-sulphamethoxazole (400/80 mg daily) to prevent PJP infection.[98]

Remission Induction of Relapsing or Refractory EGPA of Non-Life-threatening Manifestations

In EGPA, relapse signifies the return of clinical symptoms after a period of remission. It is crucial to differentiate this from mere increases in eosinophil count without accompanying clinical features.[99,100] EGPA relapses can be categorized as systemic (vasculitis) or respiratory (isolated asthma and ENT involvement).

For respiratory relapses, initial management involves topical bronchodilators and low-dose oral steroids. Unresponsive cases may warrant a short course of high-dose glucocorticoids (0.5–1 mg/kg/day for 5–7 days), followed by immediate discontinuation without tapering.[101] In persistently unresponsive cases, mepolizumab can be added. For relapsing ENT disease, functional endoscopic sinus surgery (FESS) is an option if conservative measures prove ineffective.

For systemic relapse, mepolizumab, a humanized monoclonal antibody against IL-5, emerges as a promising option. Administered subcutaneously at 300 mg every 4 weeks for 6 months alongside low-dose steroids, it can effectively control disease, reduce steroid dependence, and offer a favorable safety profile compared to traditional immunosuppressants, as shown in the MIRRA phase 3 trial.[102] Notably, the same study suggests that a lower dose of 100 mg every 4 weeks can also be effective, particularly for controlling respiratory manifestations.[103]

Maintenance of Remission of Relapsing EGPA of Non-Life-threatening and Life-threatening Manifestations

For both non-life-threatening and life-threatening relapsing EGPA, maintaining remission often relies on a combination of glucocorticoids and mepolizumab.

Treatment of EGPA in Specific Situations

Age-specific considerations are crucial. A study demonstrated that reducing cyclophosphamide dosage (500 mg fixed dose vs 500 mg/m^2) and shortening glucocorticoid treatment duration (9 vs 26 months) in patients over 65 maintained remission rates while minimizing adverse events.[104]

For EGPA patients over 65 years old, an open-label trial demonstrated that a reduced cyclophosphamide dosage (fixed 500 mg instead of 500 mg/m^2) and shorter glucocorticoid treatment (9 months instead of 26 months) could effectively lower the risk of adverse events without compromising remission rates.[105]

During pregnancy, managing EGPA requires careful consideration due to medication limitations. While glucocorticoids, intravenous immunoglobulins, and azathioprine are considered relatively safe, rituximab and mepolizumab lack sufficient safety data and should be avoided.[106] Additionally, cyclophosphamide, mycophenolate mofetil, and methotrexate are contraindicated and must be discontinued 3–6 months before conception. It is crucial to note that pregnancy loss remains a potential risk, affecting up to 20% of patients with EGPA.[107,108]

GOODPASTURE SYNDROME

Goodpasture syndrome, also known as anti-GBM disease, is a rare yet potentially life-threatening condition characterized by small vessel vasculitis. The hallmark feature lies in the presence of circulating antibodies targeting a crucial antigen: The α3 chain of type IV collagen, abundantly present in both the glomerular basement membrane (GBM) of the kidneys and the alveolar basement membrane (ABM) of the lungs. This immunological attack leads to the development of rapidly progressive glomerulonephritis (RPGN) and/or alveolar hemorrhage (DAH).[109,110]

Treatment

In Goodpasture syndrome, the core therapeutic strategy hinges on eliminating circulating anti-GBM antibodies through plasmapheresis while simultaneously halting further antibody production. This is achieved by a combination of immunosuppressive medications, primarily corticosteroids and cyclophosphamide, alongside eliminating any identified triggers.

Initial therapy includes plasmapheresis combined with immunosuppressive therapy (glucocorticoids and cyclophosphamide), except for those who are on dialysis and do not have pulmonary hemorrhage.[111] Oral prednisolone is given at 1 mg/kg/day (maximum 60 mg), followed by a gradual weekly reduction to 20 mg by 6 weeks, followed by further tapering until complete discontinuation over 6–9 months. Studies suggest better renal outcomes with combined plasmapheresis and steroids compared to steroids alone. Studies suggest better renal outcomes with combined plasmapheresis and steroids compared to steroids alone.[112,113] The Levy JB et al study suggests pulsed intravenous methylprednisolone (15–30 mg/kg to a maximum of 1000 mg over 20 minutes daily for 3 days) followed by oral prednisolone (1 mg/kg/day, maximum 60–80 mg) for up to 6 months. This regimen can be tapered once remission is achieved. McAdoo SP et al says IV methylprednisolone and IV cyclophosphamide are used for the fulminant anti-GBM disease at a few centres, though there is inadequate data to support this.[114]

Cyclophosphamide, a key component of immunosuppressive therapy for anti-GBM disease, is typically administered orally at 2 mg/kg/day for 3–6 months. This dosage is adjusted to maintain a white blood cell count of around 5000 while minimizing corticosteroid requirements. For patients achieving prompt remission, cyclophosphamide can be continued for 2–3 months and steroids for 6 months. However, those with ongoing clinical or serological activity at 3–4 months need extended immunosuppression up to 6–9 months. A Chinese study highlighted the potential benefits of combining plasmapheresis with cytotoxic and steroid therapy, suggesting a synergistic effect in achieving better outcomes.[115]

For patients with refractory anti-GBM disease unable to tolerate cyclophosphamide, rituximab (1 g × 2 doses) offers a valuable alternative. Additionally, mycophenolate mofetil and azathioprine serve as viable options to reduce adverse effects in specific cases.[116] Maintenance therapy is generally not required for anti-GBM disease. However, for patients with anti-GBM and ANCA positivity, an approach similar to ANCA-associated vasculitis (AAV) maintenance therapy may be warranted. Atypical anti-GBM disease, characterized by mild renal involvement and lack of widespread crescent formation, often does not require immunosuppression initially. However, close monitoring is crucial, and therapy can be initiated if progressive glomerulonephritis develops.[117]

RELAPSING POLYCHONDRITIS

Relapsing polychondritis (RP) presents a unique immunological challenge characterized by recurring attacks on cartilaginous and proteoglycan-rich tissues throughout the body. This progressive inflammatory/degenerative disease damages these structures, leading to functional and anatomical impairment that can manifest as ear deformities, joint pain, and even life-threatening airway issues. Although RP primarily targets cartilage, its complex nature involves both humoral and cell-mediated immune pathways. Notably, circulating autoantibodies against specific collagen types (II, IX, and XI) have been identified in RP patients, potentially contributing to the formation of immune complexes that might play a role in driving inflammatory damage.[118] Remove immune complexes bound to the surface of cartilage by scavenger cells facilitates the release of matrix-degrading metalloproteinases, oxygen metabolites and/or cytokines. Chronic inflammation causes granulation tissue and peribronchial fibrosis, leading to fixed or dynamic airway narrowing, stenosis or strictures in the subglottic airway, tracheal collapse, and secondary pulmonary infections.[119]

Treatment

Treatment aims to control inflammatory crisis with NSAIDs, corticosteroids, and immunosuppressant drugs to achieve rapid relief of symptoms and to prevent multi-organ effects on cartilaginous structures, with fewer side effects. Mild inflammatory disease includes nasal or auricular chondritis with peripheral or axial arthritis with no major organ involvement are treated with NSAIDs for 7–10 days, colchicine (1.2–2.4 mg per day in 2–4 divided doses), dapsone (50–100 mg once daily maximum of 200 mg per day), and low-dose corticosteroids, However, steroid-resistant scenarios or severe manifestations like ocular, laryngotracheal, cardiac, vasculitic, or widespread polychondritis require systemic corticosteroids, the mainstay of treatment.[120–123]

Steroid treatment and follow-up are needed to decrease the frequency, duration, and severity of relapses, but do not modify disease progression. Dose of oral prednisone 0.25–1 mg/kg/day. The glucocorticoid should be gradually tapered, as long as the disease remains under control, to a maintenance level of 5–7.5 mg daily. Medications should be reinstituted, or the dose increased when symptoms recur during this taper. The disease can be monitored clinically and by testing nonspecific inflammatory marker ESR. Once a stable dose is achieved and treatment has been maintained for three months without recurrent disease, an effort is made to further reduce and discontinue the medications.

Trachcobronchial involvement in RP, like tracheomalacia, can result in airway collapse; airway interventions like balloon dilatation, stent placement, tracheostomy, or a combination of techniques may be frequently required.[124] ReCONNET Center for RP proposed a therapeutic strategy that nasal and auricular RP mostly suffices with NSAIDs; rest all organ involvements require glucocorticoids, DMARDs, conventional immunosuppressants, or biologics. Neurological, tracheal, and audiovestibular manifestations require aggressive IV methylprednisolone therapy.[125]

If an organ or life-threatening disease like sudden sensorineural hearing loss, ocular involvement, systemic vasculitis, severe laryngotracheal chondritis, renal or neurologic involvement, high-dose systemic steroids, and immunosuppressants are required, given as pulse intravenous methyl prednisone (1 g bolus per day for three consecutive days). A combination of prednisone (usually 1 mg/kg daily) with oral cyclophosphamide (initially at 2 mg/kg daily by mouth). Prednisone should be maintained at the initial starting dose for the first month, then tapered gradually once disease activity is controlled, to 7.5 mg or less daily by six months.[126] There are no proven or formal consensus guidelines indicating how long maintenance therapy with glucocorticoids or alternative agents should be continued before attempting withdrawal.

Immunosuppressants (azathioprine 2 mg/kg/day, subsequently tapered to a maintenance level of 50–75 mg/day, and cyclosporine 5 mg/kg/day, subsequently tapered to a lower maintenance dose) are also indicated in a corticosteroid-intolerant or lack of response to steroids or the necessity of corticosteroid-sparing therapy. French multicenter retrospective study showed good response with biologics like TNF-α inhibitors, adalimumab or infliximab, tocilizumab, anakinra, rituximab, and abatacept and reduction of steroid doses was highly variable. The overall response is 62.9% in the first 6 months of the treatment.[127]

REFERENCES

1. Walker WC, Wright V. Pulmonary lesions and rheumatoid arthritis. Medicine (Baltimore). 1968;47(6):501–20.
2. Chen J, Shi Y, Wang X, et al. Asymptomatic preclinical rheumatoid arthritis-associated interstitial lung disease. Clin Dev Immunol. 2013;2013:406927.
3. Gochuico BR, Avila NA, Chow CK, Novero LJ, Wu HP, Ren P, MacDonald SD, Travis WD, Stylianou MP, Rosas IO. Progressive preclinical interstitial lung disease in rheumatoid arthritis. Arch Intern Med. 2008 Jan 28;168(2):159–66.
4. Scally SW, Petersen J, Law SC, Dudek NL, Nel HJ, Loh KL, Wijeyewickrema LC, Eckle SBG, van Heemst J, Pike RN, et al. A molecular basis for the association of the HLA-DRB1 locus, citrullination, and rheumatoid arthritis. J. Exp. Med. 2013;210:2569–82.
5. Iftikhar IH, Alghothani L, Sardi A, Berkowitz D, Musani AI Transbronchial Lung Cryobiopsy and Video-assisted Thoracoscopic Lung Biopsy in the Diagnosis of Diffuse Parenchymal Lung Disease. A Meta-analysis of Diagnostic Test Accuracy. Ann. Am. Thorac. Soc. 2017;14:1197–1211.
6. Cush JJ. Early rheumatoid arthritis is there a window of opportunity? J Rheumatol. 2007;80:1–7.
7. Combe B. Progression in early rheumatoid arthritis. Best Pract Res Clin Rheumatol. 2009;23:59–69.
8. Sizova L. Approaches to the treatment of early rheumatoid arthritis with disease-modifying antirheumatic drugs. Br J Clin Pharmacol. 2008;66:173–8.
9. Wells AU, Hirani N, on behalf of the British Thoracic Society Interstitial Lung Disease Guideline Group, a subgroup of the British Thoracic Society Standards of Care Committee, in collaboration with the Thoracic Society of Australia and New Zealand and the Irish Thoracic Society. Interstitial lung disease guideline: the British Thoracic Society in collaboration with the Thoracic Society of Australia and New Zealand and the Irish Thoracic Society. Thorax. (2008) 63(Suppl V):v1–v58. doi: 10.1136/thx.2008.101691.
10. Wijsenbeek M, Bendstrup E, Valenzuela C, Henry MT, Moor C, Bengus M, Perjesi A, Gilberg F, Kirchgaessler KU, Vancheri C. Design of a Study Assessing Disease Behaviour During the Peri-Diagnostic Period in Patients with Interstitial Lung Disease: The STARLINER Study. Adv. Ther. 2019;36:232–243. doi: 10.1007/s12325-018-0845-3.
11. Ota M, Iwasaki Y, Harada H, Sasaki O, Nagafuchi Y, Nakachi S, Sumitomo S, Shoda H, Tohma S, Fujio K, et al. Efficacy of intensive immunosuppression in exacerbated rheumatoid arthritis-associated interstitial lung disease. Mod. Rheumatol. 2017;27:22–28.doi: 10.3109/14397595.2016.1173816. [PubMed] [CrossRef] [Google Scholar].
12. Combe B, Landewe R, Daien CI, Hua C, Aletaha D, Álvaro-Gracia JM, et al. 2016 update of the EULAR recommendations for the management of early arthritis. Ann Rheum Dis. 2017 Jun;76((6)):948–59. [PubMed] [Google Scholar] [Ref list].
13. Finckh A, Liang MH, van Herckenrode CM, de Pablo P. Long-term impact of early treatment on radiographic progression in rheumatoid arthritis: A meta-analysis. Arthritis Rheum. 2006;55:864–72.
14. Svensson B, Boonen A, Albertsson K, et al. Low-dose prednisolone in addition to the initial disease-modifying antirheumatic drug in patients with early active rheumatoid arthritis reduces joint destruction and increases the remission rate: a two-year randomized trial. Arthritis Rheum. 2005;52:3360–70.
15. Hafström I, Albertsson K, Boonen A, et al. Remission achieved after 2 years of treatment with low-dose prednisolone in addition to disease-modifying anti-rheumatic drugs in early rheumatoid arthritis is associated with reduced joint destruction still present after 4 years: an open 2-year continuation study. Ann Rheum Dis. 2009;68(4):508–13.

16. Kirwan JR, Bijlsma JW, Boers M, Shea BJ. Effects of glucocorticoids on radiological progression in rheumatoid arthritis. Cochrane Database Syst Rev. 2007 [PMC free article] [PubMed] [Google Scholar] [Ref list].
17. Puechal X, Gottenberg JE, Berthelot JM, et al. Rituximab therapy for systemic vasculitis associated with rheumatoid arthritis: results from the AutoImmunity and Rituximab Registry. Arthritis Care Res (Hoboken). 2012;64(3):331–39.
18. Geddes DM, Corrin B, Brewerton DA, et al. Progressive airway obliteration in adults and its association with rheumatoid disease. Q J Med. 1977;46(184):427–44.
19. Devouassoux G, Cottin V, Liote H, et al. Characterisation of severe obliterative bronchiolitis in rheumatoid arthritis. Eur Respir J. 2009;33(5):1053–61.
20. Shin JI, Lee KH, Park S, Yang JW, Kim HJ, Song K, Lee S, Na H, Jang YJ, Nam JY, et al. Systemic Lupus Erythematosus and Lung Involvement: A Comprehensive Review. J. Clin. Med. 2022;11:6714. doi: 10.3390/jcm11226714.
21. Lian FZJ, Wang Y, Cui W, Chen D, Li H, Qiu Q, et al. Clinical features and independent predictors of interstitial lung disease in systemic lupus erythematosus. Int J Clin Exp Med. (2016) 9:4233–42].
22. Fanouriakis A, Kostopoulou M, Alunno A, Aringer M, Bajema I, Boletis JN, Cervera R, Doria A, Gordon C, Govoni M, et al. 2019 Update of the EULAR Recommendations for the Management of Systemic Lupus Erythematosus. Ann. Rheum. Dis. 2019;78:736–745. doi: 10.1136/annrheumdis-2019-215089.
23. Lee CT, Strek ME. The Other Connective Tissue Disease-associated Interstitial Lung Diseases: Sjogren's Syndrome, Mixed Connective Tissue Disease, and Systemic Lupus Erythematosus. Curr. Opin. Pulm. Med. 2021;27:388–95.
24. Muangchan C, van Vollenhoven RF Bernatsky SR, Smith CD, Hudson M, Inanç M, Rothfield NF, Nash PT, Furie RA, Senécal JL, et al. Treatment Algorithms in Systemic Lupus Erythematosus. Arthritis Care Res. 2015;67:1237–1245. doi: 10.1002/acr.22589.
25. Vacchi C, Sebastiani M, Cassone G, Cerri S, Della Casa G, Salvarani C, Manfredi A. Therapeutic Options for the Treatment of Interstitial Lung Disease Related to Connective Tissue Diseases. A Narrative Review. J. Clin. Med. 2020;9:407.
26. Koo SM, Uh ST. Treatment of Connective Tissue Disease-associated Interstitial Lung Disease: The Pulmonologist's Point of View. Korean J. Intern. Med. 2017;32:600–610. doi: 10.3904/kjim.2016.212.
27. Weinrib L, Sharma OP, Quismorio FP. A Long-Term Study of Interstitial Lung Disease in Systemic Lupus Erythematosus. Semin. Arthritis Rheum. 1990;20:48–56.
28. Roca F, Dominique S, Schmidt J, Smail A, Duhaut P, Lévesque H, Marie I. Interstitial lung disease in primary Sjögren's syndrome. Autoimmun. Rev. 2017;16:48–54. doi: 10.1016/j.autrev.2016.09.017.
29. Robles-Perez A., Molina-Molina M. Treatment Considerations of Lung Involvement in Rheumatologic Disease. Respiration. 2015;90:265–74.
30. Fishman's Pulmonary Diseases and Disorders 6th edition.
31. Rahaghi FF, Hsu VM, Kaner RJ, et al. Expert consensus on the management of systemic sclerosis-associated interstitial lung disease. Respir Res 2023;24(6):
32. Murray & Nadel's textbook of Respiratory Medicine 7th edition.
33. Cappelli S, Bellando Randone S, Camiciottoli G, De Paulis A, Guiducci S, Matucci-Cerinic M. Interstitial lung disease in systemic sclerosis: where do we stand? Eur Respir Rev. 2015 Sep;24(137):411–9.
34. Tashkin DP, Elashoff R, Clements PJ, et al. Cyclophosphamide versus placebo in scleroderma lung disease. N Engl J Med. 2006;354:2655–66.
35. Tashkin DP, Roth MD, Clements PJ, et al. Mycophenolate mofetil versus oral cyclophosphamide in scleroderma-related interstitial lung disease (SLS II): a randomised controlled, double-blind, parallel-group trial. Lancet Respir Med. 2016;4:708–19.
36. Ando K, Motojima S, Doi T, et al. Effect of glucocorticoid monotherapy on pulmonary function and survival in Japanese patients with scleroderma-related interstitial lung disease. Respir Invest 2013;51:69–75.

37. Steen VD, Medsger TA, Jr. Case-control study of corticosteroids and other drugs that either precipitate or protect from the development of scleroderma renal crisis. Arthritis Rheum. 1998;41:1613–19.
38. Herrick AL. Controversies on the use of steroids in systemic sclerosis. J Scleroderma Relat Disord 2017;2:84–91.
39. Griffiths-Jones DJ, Garcia YS, Ryder WD, Pauling JD, Hall FL, et al. A Phase II randomized controlled trial of oral prednisolone in early diffuse cutaneous systemic sclerosis (PRedSS). Rheumatology (Oxford). 2023 Sep 1;62(9):3133–38.
40. Lorrain Thong1. Liam J. Chawke2. Grainne Murphy3. Michael T. Henry 4 Management of myositis associated interstitial lung disease May 2023.
41. Barba T, Fort R, Cottin V, Provencher S, Durieu I, Jardel S, Hot A, Reynaud Q, Lega JC, Treatment of idiopathic inflammatory myosotis associated interstitial lung disease: A systematic review and metaanalysis. Autoimmun Rev. 2019.
42. Lundberg IE, Tjärnlund A, Bottai M, Werth VP, Pilkington C, Visser M, Alfredsson L, Amato AA, Barohn RJ, Liang MH et al 2017 European League Against Rheumatism/American College of Rheumatology classification criteria for adult and juvenile idiopathic inflammatory myopathies and their major subgroups. Ann. Rheum. Dis. 2017;76:1955–64.
43. Hallowell RW, Danoff SK. Diagnosis and Management of Myositis-associated Lung Disease. Chest. 2023 Feb 9.
44. T Minura, H Kanda, K Kubo, Treatment of steroid-resistant polymyositis and dermatomyositis. Ni hon Rinsho. 2001 Oct;59(10):2062–70.
45. Simone Baesotti, Ingrid E. Lundberg, Current Treatment of Myositis, Curr Treatm Opt Rheumatol. 2018;4(4):299–315.
46. Serena Fasano, Patrick Gordon, Raouf Hajji, Esthela Loyo, David A. Isenberg Rheumatology, Rituximab in the treatment of inflammatory myopathies: a review, Rheumatology, January 2017; 56(1):26–36.
47. Kurita T, Yasuda S, Oba K, et al. The efficacy of tacrolimus in patients with interstitial lung diseases complicated with polymyositis or dermatomyositis. Rheumatology (Oxford) 2015;54(1):39–44.
48. Wallace B, Vummidi D, Khanna D. Management of connective tissue diseases associated interstitial lung disease: A review of the published literature. Curr. Opin. Rheumatol. 2016;28:236–45.
49. Ingegnoli F, Lubatti C, Ingegnoli A, Boracchi P, Zeni S, Meroni PL. Interstitial lung disease outcomes by high-resolution computed tomography (HRCT) in Anti-Jo1 antibody-positive polymyositis patients: A single centre study and review of the literature. Autoimmun. Rev. 2012;11:335–40.
50. Chen IJ, Jan Wu YJ, Lin CW, Fan KW, Luo SF, Ho HH. Interstitial lung disease in polymyositis and dermatomyositis. Clin. Rheumatol. 2009;28:639–46.
51. Hozumi H, Fujisawa T, Nakashima R, Yasui H, Suzuki Y, Kono M, Karayama M, Furuhashi K, Enomoto N, Inui N, et al. Efficacy of Glucocorticoids and Calcineurin Inhibitors for Anti-aminoacyl-tRNA Synthetase Antibody-positive Polymyositis/ dermatomyositis-associated Interstitial Lung Disease: A Propensity Score-matched Analysis. J.Rheumatol. 2019;46:509–17.
52. Reiseter S, Gunnarsson R, Corander J, Haydon J, Lund MB, Aaløkken TM, Taraldsrud E, Hetlevik SO, Molberg Ø. Disease evolution in mixed connective tissue disease: Results from a long-term nationwide prospective cohort study. Arthritis Res. Ther. 2017;21:284.
53. Hoffman GS, Kerr GS, Leavitt RY, et al. Wegener granulomatosis: An analysis of 158 patients. Ann Intern Med. 1992;116(6):488–98.
54. Cartin-Ceba R, Peikert T, Specks U. Pathogenesis of ANCA associated vasculitis. Curr Rheumatol Rep. 2012;14(6):481–93.
55. Hervier B, Pagnoux C, Agard C, Haroche J, Amoura Z, Guillevin L, et al. Vasculitis study, pulmonary fibrosis associated with ANCA-positive vasculitides. Retrospective study of 12 cases and review of the literature. Ann Rheum Dis 2009;68:404–7.
56. Antonelou M, Abro A, Heath R, et al. Comparison of outcomes using the rituximab originator MabThera with the biosimilar truxima in patients with ANCA-associated vasculitis. Scand J Rheumatol 2022;51:135–41.

57. De Groot K, Rasmussen N, Bacon PA, et al. Randomized trial of cyclophosphamide versus methotrexate for induction of remission in early systemic antineutrophil cytoplasmic antibody-associated vasculitis. Arthritis Rheum 2005;52:2461–9.
58. Faurschou, M, et al. Brief report: long-term outcome of a randomized clinical trial comparing methotrexate to cyclophosphamide for remission induction in early systemic antineutrophil cytoplasmic antibody-associated vasculitis. Arthritis Rheumatol. 2012;64:3472–77.
59. Smith RM, Jones RB, Specks U, et al. Rituximab as therapy to induce remission after relapse in ANCA-associated vasculitis. Ann Rheum Dis 2020;79:1243–9.
60. Jayne DRW, Merkel PA, Schall TJ, et al. Avacopan for the treatment of ANCA-associated vasculitis. *N Engl J Med* 2021;384:599–609.
61. Jayne, DRW. et al. Randomized trial of C5a receptor inhibitor avacopan in ANCA-associated vasculitis. *J. Am. Soc. Nephrol.* 2017;28:2756–67.
62. Merkel, PA. et al. A randomised, double-blind, active-controlled study of Avacopan in anti-neutrophil cytoplasmic antibody (ANCA)-associated vasculitis. Ann. Rheum. Dis. 2020;79:8.
63. Merkel PA, Jayne DR, Wang C, Hillson J and Bekker P. Evaluation of the safety and efficacy of avacopan, a C5a receptor inhibitor, in patients with antineutrophil cytoplasmic antibody-associated vasculitis treated concomitantly with rituximab or cyclophosphamide/azathioprine: protocol for a randomized, double-blind, active-controlled, Phase 3 trial. JMIR Res. Protoc. 2020;9:e16664.
64. Jayne D, Rasmussen N, Andrassy K, et al. A randomized trial of maintenance therapy for vasculitis associated with antineutrophil cytoplasmic autoantibodies. *N Engl J Med* 2003;349:36–44.
65. Levy JB, Turner AN, Rees AJ, et al. Long-term outcome of anti-glomerular basement membrane antibody disease treated with plasma exchange and immunosuppression. Ann Intern Med 2001;134:1033–42.
66. Gopaluni S, et al. Effect of disease activity at three and six months after diagnosis on long-term outcomes in antineutrophil cytoplasmic antibody-associated vasculitis. Arthritis Rheumatol 2019;71:784–91.
67. Walsh M, et al. Plasma exchange and glucocorticoids in severe ANCA-associated vasculitis. *N. Engl. J. Med.* 2020;382:622–631. A clinical trial of induction therapies in severe AAV, demonstrates that lower-dose glucocorticoids are non-inferior to standard doses and that routine use of plasma exchange as an adjuvant provides no additional benefit.
68. Garlapati P, Qurie A. Granulomatosis With Polyangiitis. 2022 Dec 5. In: StatPearls [Internet]. Treasure Island (FL): StatPearls Publishing; 2023 Jan–. PMID: 32491759.
69. Stone JH, Merkel PA, Spiera R, et al. Rituximab versus cyclophosphamide for ANCA-associated vasculitis. N Engl J Med 2010;363:221–32.
70. Guillevin L, Pagnoux C, Karras A, et al. Rituximab versus azathioprine for maintenance in ANCA-associated vasculitis. *N Engl J Med* 2014;371:1771–80.
71. Charles P, Perrodeau É, Samson M, et al. Long-term rituximab use to maintain remission of antineutrophil cytoplasmic antibody-associated vasculitis: a randomized trial. Ann Intern Med 2020;173:179–87.
72. Charles P, Terrier B, Perrodeau É, et al. Comparison of individually tailored versus fixed-schedule rituximab regimen to maintain ANCA-associated vasculitis remission: results of a multicentre, randomised controlled, phase III trial (MAINRITSAN2). Ann Rheum Dis 2018;77:1143–9.
73. Smith R, Jayne D and Merkel P. A randomized, controlled trial of rituximab versus azathioprine after induction of remission with rituximab for patients with ANCA-associated vasculitis and relapsing disease (abstract). Arthritis Rheumatol. 71 (Suppl. 10) (2019).
74. Gopaluni S, et al. Rituximab versus azathioprine as therapy for maintenance of remission for antineutrophil cytoplasm antibody-associated vasculitis (RITAZAREM): study protocol for a randomized controlled trial. Trials 2017;18:112.
75. Kitching AR, Anders HJ, Basu N, et al. ANCA-associated vasculitis.Nat Rev Dis Primers. 2020;6(1):71.
76. Foulon G, Delaval P, Valeyre D, Wallaert B, Debray MP, Brauner M, et al. ANCA-associated lung fibrosis: analysis of 17 patients. Respir Med.

77. Homma S, Matsushita H, Nakata K. Pulmonary fibrosis in myeloperoxidase antineutrophil cytoplasmic antibody-associated vasculitides. Respirology 2004;9:190–6.
78. Ando M, Miyazaki E, Ishii T, Mukai Y, Yamasue M, Fujisaki H, et al. Incidence of myeloperoxidase anti-neutrophil cytoplasmic antibody positivity and microscopic polyangiitis in the course of idiopathic pulmonary fibrosis. Respir Med 2013;107:608–15.
79. Jayne DR, et al. Intravenous immunoglobulin for ANCA-associated systemic vasculitis with persistent disease activity. QJM 2000;93:433–39.
80. Churg JC, Strauss L. Allergic granulomatosis, allergic angiitis and periarteritis nodosa. Am J Pathol. 1951;27(2):277–301.
81. Jakiela B, Sanak M, Szczeklik W, et al. Both Th2 and Th17 responses are involved in the pathogenesis of Churg-Strauss syndrome. Clin Exp Rheumatol. 2011;29(1 suppl 64):S23–34.
82. Vaglio A, Martorana D, Maggiore U, et al. HLA-DRB4 as a genetic risk factor for Churg-Strauss syndrome. Arthritis Rheum. 2007;56(9):3159–66.
83. Wieczorek S, Hellmich B, Arning L, et al. Functionally relevant variations of the interleukin-10 gene associated with antineutrophil cytoplasmic antibody-negative Churg-Strauss syndrome, but not with Wegener's granulomatosis. Arthritis Rheum. 2008;58(6):1839–48.
84. Boita M, Guida G, Circosta P, et al. The molecular and functional characterization of clonally expanded CD8+ TCR BV T cells in eosinophilic granulomatosis with polyangiitis (EGPA). Clin Immunol. 2014;152(1-2):152–63.
85. Horai Y, Miyamura T, Takahama S, et al. Churg-Strauss syndrome is associated with elevated levels of serum interleukin-5 and T cell receptor-Cβ gene rearrangement. Mod Rheumatol. 2011; 21(1):76–8.
86. Rich AR. The role of hypersensitivity in periarteritis nodosa as indicated by seven cases developing during serum sickness and sulfonamide therapy. Bull Johns Hopkins Hosp. 1942;71:123–41.
87. Roger A, Groh M, Lorillon G, et al. Eosinophilic granulomatosis with polyangiitis (Churg-Strauss) induced by immune checkpoint inhibitors. Ann Rheum Dis. 2019;78(8):e82.
88. Nathani N, Little MA, Kunst H, Wilson D, Thickett DR. Churg-Strauss syndrome and leukotriene antagonist use: a respiratory perspective. Thorax. 2008;63(10):883–88.
89. Guillevin L, Pagnoux C, Seror R, et al. The five-factor score revisited: assessment of prognoses of systemic necrotizing vasculitides based on the French Vasculitis Study Group (FVSG) cohort. Medicine (Baltimore) 2011;90:19–27.
90. Puechal X, Pagnoux C, Baron G, et al. Adding azathioprine to remission-induction glucocorticoids for eosinophilic granulomatosis with polyangiitis (Churg-Strauss), microscopic polyangiitis, or polyarteritis nodosa without poor prognosis factors: A randomized, controlled trial. Arthritis Rheumatol 2017;69:2175–86.
91. Ribi C, et al. Treatment of Churg-Strauss syndrome without poor-prognosis factors: a multicenter, prospective, randomized, open-label study of seventy-two patients. Arthritis Rheum. 2008;58:586–94.
92. Terrier B, Pugnet G, deC, et al. Rituximab versus conventional therapeutic strategy for remission induction in eosinophilic granulomatosis with polyangiitis: A double- blind, randomized, controlled trial [abstract]. Arthritis and Rheumatology 2021;73.
93. Cohen P, et al. Churg-Strauss syndrome with poor-prognosis factors: a prospective multicenter trial comparing glucocorticoids and six or twelve cyclophosphamide pulses in forty-eight patients. Arthritis Care Res. 2007;57:686–93.
94. Contro G, et al. Neutrophil infiltrates and eosinophil aggregates in chronic rhinosinusitis with nasal polyps and EGPA. Clin. Rheumatol 2021;40:1949–57.
95. Papo M, et al. Significance of PR3-ANCA positivity in eosinophilic granulomatosis with polyangiitis (Churg-Strauss). Rheumatology 2021;60:4355–60.
96. Puéchal X, et al. Non-severe eosinophilic granulomatosis with polyangiitis: long-term outcomes after remission-induction trial. Rheumatology 2019;58:2107–16.

97. Wijetilleka S, Jayne DR, Mukhtyar C, et al. Recommendations for the management of secondary hypogammaglobulinaemia due to B cell-targeted therapies in autoimmune rheumatic diseases. Rheumatology (Oxford) 2019;58:889–96.
98. Kronbichler A, Kerschbaum J, Gopaluni S, et al. Trimethoprim-Sulfamethoxazole prophylaxis prevents severe/life-threatening infections following rituximab in antineutrophil cytoplasm antibody-associated vasculitis. Ann Rheum Dis 2018;77:1440–7.
99. Chung SA, et al. 2021 American College of Rheumatology/Vasculitis Foundation Guideline for the Management of Antineutrophil Cytoplasmic Antibody-Associated Vasculitis. Arthritis Care Res. 2021;73:1088–1105.
100. Terrier B, et al. French recommendations for the management of systemic necrotizing vasculitides (polyarteritis nodosa and ANCA-associated vasculitides). Orphanet J. Rare Dis. 15, 351 (2020).
101. Emmi G, Bettiol, A, Gelain, E, et al. Evidence-based Guideline for the diagnosis and management of eosinophilic granulomatosis with polyangiitis. Nat Rev Rheumatol 2023;19:378–393. https://doi.org/10.1038/s41584-023-00958-w.
102. Wechsler ME, Akuthota P, Jayne D, et al. Mepolizumab or placebo for eosinophilic granulomatosis with polyangiitis. N Engl J Med 2017;376:1921–32.
103. Bettiol A, et al. Mepolizumab for eosinophilic granulomatosis with polyangiitis (EGPA): a European multicenter observational study. Arthritis Rheumatol 2022;74:295–306.
104. Latorre M, et al. Asthma control and airway inflammation in patients with eosinophilic granulomatosis with polyangiitis. J. Allergy Clin. Immunol. Pract 2016;4:512–19.
105. Pagnoux C, et al. Treatment of systemic necrotizing vasculitides in patients aged sixty five years or older: results of a multicenter, open-label, randomized controlled trial of corticosteroid and cyclophosphamide-based induction therapy. Arthritis Rheumatol 2015;67:1117–27.
106. Pagnoux C, Mahendira D and Laskin CA, Fertility and pregnancy in vasculitis. Best. Pract. Res. Clin. Rheumatol. 2013;27:79–94.
107. European Medicines Agency. Nucala. https://www.ema.europa.eu/en/medicines/human/ EPAR/ nucala (2015).
108. EMA. MABTHERA-EMA. https://www.ema.europa.eu/en/medicines/human/EPAR/ mabthera (2018).
109. McAdoo SP, Pusey CD. Anti-Glomerular Basement Membrane Disease. *Clin J Am Soc Nephrol* 2017;12:1162.
110. Pedchenko V, Vanacore R, Hudson B. Goodpasture's disease: the molecular architecture of the autoantigen provides clues to aetiology and pathogenesis. Curr Opin Nephrol Hypertens. 2011;20(3):290–96.
111. Levy JB, Turner AN, Rees AJ, Pusey CD. Long-term outcome of anti-glomerular basement membrane antibody disease treated with plasma exchange and immunosuppression. Ann Intern Med 2001; 134:1033.
112. Pusey CD: Anti-glomerular basement membrane disease. Kidney Int 64: 1535–1550, 2003 [PubMed] [Google Scholar] [Ref list].
113. Johnson JP, Jr MJ, Austin HA 3rd, Balow JE, Antonovych TT, Wilson CB. Therapy of anti-glomerular basement membrane antibody disease: analysis of the prognostic significance of clinical, pathologic and treatment factors. Medicine. 1985;64(4):219–227. doi: 10.1097/00005792-198507000-00003 [PubMed] [CrossRef] [Google Scholar] [Ref list].
114. McAdoo SP, Pusey CD. Anti-glomerular basement membrane disease. *Clin J Am Soc Nephrol.* 2017;12(7):1162–1172. doi: 10.2215/CJN.01380217.
115. Cui Z, Zhao J, Jia XY, Zhu SN, Jin QZ, Cheng XY, Zhao MH: Anti-glomerular basement membrane disease: Outcomes of different therapeutic regimens in a large single-centre Chinese cohort study. Medicine (Baltimore) 2011;90:303–11.
116. Syeda UA, Singer NG, Magrey M. Anti-glomerular basement membrane antibody disease treated with rituximab: A case-based review. Semin Arthritis Rheum 2013;42:567.
117. Kaplan AA, Appel GB, Pusey CE, et al. Anti-GBM (Goodpasture) disease: treatment and prognosis. Update: evidence-based clinical decision support. Available from: www.uptodate.com. Accessed February 25, 2022. [Ref list].

118. Petitdemange, et al. Treatment of relapsing polychondritis: a systemic review. Clin Exp Rheumatol 2022;40 (Suppl.134):S81–85.
119. Eng J, Sabanathan S. Airway complications in relapsing polychondritis. Ann. Thorac. Surg. 1991;51:686–92.
120. McAdam LP, O'Hanlan MA, Bluestone R, Pearson CM. Relapsing polychondritis: a prospective study of 23 patients and a review of the literature. Medicine (Baltimore) 1976;55:193.
121. Damiani JM, Levine HL. Relapsing polychondritis—report of ten cases. Laryngoscope 1979;89:929.
122. Schumacher S, Pieringer H, Relapsing polychondritis: A chameleon among orphan diseases. Wien. Med. Wochenschr. 2017;167:227–33. [CrossRef] [PubMed].
123. Mathian A, Miyara M, Cohen-Aubart F, Haroche J, Hie M, Pha M, Grenier P, Amoura Z. Relapsing polychondritis: A 2016 update on clinical features, diagnostic tools, treatment and biological drug use. Best Pract. Res. Clin. Rheumatol. 2016;30:316–33. [CrossRef] [PubMed].
124. Ernst A, Rafeq S, Boiselle P, Sung A, Reddy C, Michaud G, Majid A, Herth FJ, Trentham D. Relapsing polychondritis and airway involvement. Chest 2009;135:1024–1030. [CrossRef] [PubMed].
125. Relapsing polychondritis: state of the art on clinical practice guidelines.Rednic S, et al. RMD Open 2018;4:e000788. doi:10.1136/rmdopen-2018-000788.
126. Smylie A, Malhotra N, Brassard A, Relapsing Polychondritis: A Review and Guide for the Dermatologist. Am. J. Clin. Dermatol. 2017;18:77–86.
127. Moulis G, Pugnet G, Costedoat-Chalumeau N, et al. Efficacy and safety of biologics in relapsing polychondritis: a French national multicentre study. Ann Rheum Dis 2018;77:1172.

Chapter

8

Steroids in Lung Infections

G Uma Sri • M Ramakrishna Reddy

Lung infections, caused by a diverse range of bacteria, viruses, and fungi, pose a significant health concern. While antibiotics remain the mainstay of therapy for bacterial infections, the use of corticosteroids in managing lung infections has become a topic of ongoing debate. This chapter delves into the intricate interplay between corticosteroids and the immune response in the context of lung infections. We will explore the potential benefits of corticosteroids, such as mitigating excessive inflammation and minimizing lung injury. However, we will also critically examine the potential drawbacks, including immunosuppression and hindering the body's ability to clear pathogens. Furthermore, we will discuss the specific applications and current evidence for corticosteroids in various lung infections, including community-acquired pneumonia (CAP), influenza pneumonia, COVID-19 pneumonia, *Pneumocystis jirovecii* pneumonia (PCP), and allergic bronchopulmonary aspergillosis (ABPA). By critically evaluating the latest research and clinical guidelines, this chapter aims to provide healthcare professionals with a comprehensive understanding of the evolving role of corticosteroids in managing lung infections, including the potential benefits, limitations, and associated risks.

COMMUNITY-ACQUIRED PNEUMONIA (CAP)

Despite medical advancements, community-acquired pneumonia (CAP) remains a prevalent disease with significant morbidity and mortality. Notably, the World Health Organization ranks lower respiratory infections as the leading infectious cause of mortality worldwide.[1] Community-acquired pneumonia can be caused by various bacterial and non-bacterial pathogens. Common bacterial culprits include *Streptococcus pneumoniae* and *Haemophilus influenzae*. *Legionella pneumophila*, associated with aspiration of contaminated water, and *Pneumocystis jirovecii*, opportunistic in immunocompromised individuals, deserve special mention. Susceptibility to these pathogens is influenced by age, underlying health conditions (comorbidities), vaccination status, immunosuppressive medication use, smoking history, recent hospitalization, and travel history.

Pneumonia pathogenesis requires microbial access to the alveoli through inhalation, aspiration, or hematogenous spread. Alveolar infiltration by microbes triggers macrophage-mediated phagocytosis. Incomplete clearance leads to an escalated immune response characterized by proinflammatory cytokine release (IL-1β, IL-6, TNF-α, IL-8). While crucial for pathogen control, this local inflammatory response unfortunately damages lung tissue, causing dyspnea, cough, sputum production, and chest pain. Insufficient local control triggers systemic cytokine release, leading to fever, tachycardia, and leukocytosis. Dysregulated systemic inflammation can spiral into severe complications like bacteremia, sepsis, ARDS, multiorgan failure, and death.

Mechanism of Corticosteroids in CAP

The exact mechanism of corticosteroids in CAP remains highly debated. Several proposed mechanisms offer potential explanations for their benefits, but conclusive evidence is lacking. One theory centres around their anti-inflammatory properties. They might downregulate proinflammatory cytokines and inhibit immune cell migration, potentially reducing inflammation and preventing respiratory failure in severe cases. Another hypothesis suggests they normalize the hypothalamus-pituitary-adrenal axis (HPA axis) in patients with inadequate adrenal response due to critical illness, similar to their role in septic shock. Additionally, corticosteroids might prevent Jarisch-Herxheimer-like reactions when initiating antibiotics in patients with high bacterial loads.[2] However, despite these theoretical advantages, the clinical efficacy of corticosteroids in CAP remains uncertain.

Literature Review and Rationale

Extensive clinical trial and meta-analysis investigations over the past two decades have yielded conflicting results regarding the role of corticosteroids in CAP management, with some demonstrating potential benefit and others suggesting harm. Corticosteroids' role in CAP remains nuanced. While Stern et al, 2017 meta-analysis across 17 RCTs demonstrated a mortality benefit in severe CAP (2264 participants), no such advantage was seen in nonsevere cases.[3] Additionally, corticosteroids shortened the time to clinical resolution, hospital/ICU stays, and late-onset respiratory failure/shock. Similarly, Briel et al, 2018 analysis of 6 RCTs with hospitalized CAP patients showed improved clinical stability and shorter hospital stays with adjunctive corticosteroids but no significant mortality effect.[4] These findings suggest potential benefits for specific CAP subsets, like reducing morbidity and aiding resolution, but underscore the need for cautious individualization due to the lack of consistent mortality benefits across all severities.

In Confalonieri's study on severe CAP, hydrocortisone (200 mg bolus followed by 10 mg/hour for 7 days) significantly improved outcomes compared to placebo in 48 patients. By day 8, the corticosteroid group showed enhanced oxygenation (PaO_2/FiO_2), improved chest X-ray scores, and reduced incidence of delayed septic shock, hospital stay, and ICU/hospital mortality.[5] This suggests the potential benefits of corticosteroids in specific severe CAP subsets, warranting further investigation. ESCAPE and CAPE COD, two randomized trials exploring corticosteroids in severe CAP, reveal conflicting results. While ESCAPE saw no mortality benefit with methylprednisolone, CAPE COD showed hydrocortisone significantly reduced 28-day mortality.[6,7] These discrepancies warrant cautious interpretation. Differences in patient demographics (ESCAPE's 96% male vs CAPE COD's 69% male) and timing of administration (CAPE COD within 24 hours vs ESCAPE up to 96 hours) likely played a role. Steroids' effects on inflammation differ across its phases, highlighting the need for further research on optimal timing and patient tailoring in this complex therapeutic landscape. While definitive corticosteroid regimens for CAP remain undefined, evidence from past trials indicates various options, including daily prednisone doses of 40–50 mg or 0.5 mg/kg/day methylprednisolone for 5–7 days. Additional studies are needed to establish optimal dosing and duration.[6,7]

Current Guideline Recommendations for Corticosteroid use in CAP

The 2007 IDSA/ATS guidelines on CAP management avoided definitive statements about corticosteroid use.[8] Despite the potential benefits of corticosteroids, the 2019 IDSA/ATS guidelines take a cautious stance on their use in CAP. This update discouraged routine use of corticosteroids in both non-severe and severe CAP cases, including influenza pneumonia. However, the guidelines align with the Surviving Sepsis Campaign recommendations, endorsing the use of corticosteroids in CAP patients with septic shock unresponsive to standard fluid resuscitation and vasopressor support.[9] The use of corticosteroids in severe CAP requiring ICU care remains a complex decision. The 2017 South African guidelines suggest considering them (e.g. methylprednisolone 0.5 mg/kg/12 hours) unless influenza, tuberculosis, or recent gastrointestinal bleeding is suspected.[10] However, the 2023 ERS/ESICM/ESCMID/ALAT guidelines suggest corticosteroid use in severe community-acquired pneumonia (sCAP) patients with shock. This recommendation does not apply to those with viral sCAP etiologies (influenza, SARS, MERS), uncontrolled diabetes, or existing corticosteroid therapy for other reasons. Methylprednisolone (0.5 mg/kg every 12 hours for 5 days) is a recommended option when considering corticosteroids.[11]

Conclusion

In conclusion, the use of corticosteroids for community-acquired pneumonia (CAP) remains a complex issue. While some studies suggest potential benefits, particularly for reducing complications and shortening hospital stays in severe cases, there is no clear evidence of mortality reduction across all CAP severities. The risk of increased infections with corticosteroids necessitates cautious use. Current guidelines advise against routine steroid use but acknowledge their potential value in severe CAP patients with septic shock unresponsive to other treatments. Early administration (within 24 hours) of corticosteroids like prednisone (40–50 mg/day) or methylprednisolone (0.5 mg/kg/day) for 5–7 days might be considered in such cases, but further research is needed.

INFLUENZA PNEUMONIA

Influenza A and B are RNA viruses belonging to the Orthomyxoviridae family that frequently cause severe clinical presentations like pneumonia and ARDS. Types A and B are the primary human influenza viruses, with type A causing yearly epidemics and pandemics due to its ability to undergo antigenic drift and shift. The major causes of ALI and ARDS following H1N1 influenza infection include cell death in the pulmonary parenchyma due to apoptosis of epithelial cells and exaggerated inflammation during infection, leading to high morbidity and mortality. Given the severity of these conditions, corticosteroids have been explored as potential adjunctive therapy. However, the efficacy and safety of this approach remain a subject of ongoing debate.

The first multicenter observational study in 2011, encompassing 220 intensive care unit (ICU) patients, raised concerns about potential downsides. It found an association between corticosteroid use and increased ICU mortality, as well as a higher risk of hospital-acquired pneumonia.[12] Other studies, such as the one by Diaz et al, further supported the lack of survival benefit from corticosteroid therapy.[13] Conversely, Brun-Buisson et al[14] suggested that very early administration of corticosteroids could be detrimental in ARDS secondary to influenza pneumonia.[14]

The 2019 IDSA/ATS pneumonia guidelines advise against routine corticosteroid use in adults with severe influenza pneumonia, citing low-quality evidence and potential risks. Furthermore, a large meta-analysis analyzing over 6,500 patients revealed higher mortality rates in those treated with corticosteroids.[15] While some studies suggest potential benefits in specific contexts, like low-dose therapy for severe hypoxia, the overall picture leans towards caution. The timing of administration also seems crucial, with potential risks associated with early initiation in ARDS patients.

An overwhelming majority of studies investigating corticosteroids for severe influenza pneumonia have yielded disappointing results. Not only did they fail to demonstrate any clinically significant benefits, but they also revealed potential downsides. Patients treated with corticosteroids experienced an increased risk of mortality, a higher incidence of hospital-acquired pneumonia (HAP), and prolonged stays in the intensive care unit (ICU), highlighting the need for caution in this context. Overall, the use of corticosteroids in influenza-related pneumonia/ARDS remains a complex issue with conflicting evidence. Further research with clear inclusion criteria, adjusted analyses, and well-designed clinical trials is crucial for definitive conclusions and optimal treatment strategies.

Conclusion

In conclusion, the use of corticosteroids for influenza pneumonia is strongly discouraged by current guidelines due to a lack of proven benefits and potential for harm. Studies overwhelmingly show no improvement in mortality rates, and even suggest increased risks like hospital-acquired pneumonia and longer ICU stays with steroid use. While some studies propose potential benefits in specific situations, the overall evidence leans towards caution. The timing of administration also seems critical, with potential downsides associated with early use. Further well-designed clinical trials are necessary to explore any specific contexts where corticosteroids might be beneficial in influenza pneumonia, but for now, they are not recommended as a routine treatment.

STEROIDS IN COVID-19 PNEUMONIA

In late 2019, a novel coronavirus (2019-nCoV) emerged in Wuhan, China, causing an atypical pneumonia. The virus utilizes angiotensin-converting enzyme 2 (ACE2) on airway epithelial cells, primarily type II alveolar cells, to initiate infection. Binding occurs via the S1 subunit's receptor-binding domain, initiating an immune response involving monocytes, T cells, B cells, and natural killer cells, leading to cytokine and chemokine release. This triggers a massive influx of inflammatory cells into the lungs, and an overactive immune response ("cytokine storm") can inflict further lung damage. Notably, compared to SARS-CoV-1, peak viral replication in 2019-nCoV occurs early, often within the first few days, while peak viral shedding declines thereafter.[16] However, around the second week, the host's inflammatory response takes centre stage, potentially leading to ARDS, multi-organ failure, and coagulation disorders.

Corticosteroids exert their effects on COVID-19 pneumonia by dampening the inflammatory response, primarily through blocking cytokine release and suppressing T cell activity. However, concerns arose from past studies on SARS and MERS, where corticosteroids showed no survival benefit but potentially hindered viral clearance and caused adverse effects. Consequently, the WHO initially advised against their routine use in COVID-19, except for specific situations like ARDS, asthma, and COPD exacerbations. Notably, no evidence supports using corticosteroids in nonhospitalized patients with COVID-19, highlighting the need for further research to determine their safety and efficacy in this population.

The RECOVERY trial, a large-scale UK study, established that dexamethasone (6 mg daily for 10 days) reduced 28-day mortality in hospitalized COVID-19 patients requiring supplemental oxygen or mechanical ventilation. However, no benefit was observed in patients who did not need oxygen support.[17] However, questions arose regarding potentially higher benefits with increased doses. Subsequent trials like COVID STEROID 2 (12 mg vs 6 mg dexamethasone) and COVIDISCUS (20 mg dexamethasone) showed mixed results. The COVID STEROID 2 trial, comparing 6 mg and 12 mg of dexamethasone in ventilated or high-flow oxygen patients, found no difference in ventilator-free days.[18] Similarly, the COVIDISCUS trial, comparing 20 mg dexamethasone with standard care in patients with severe hypoxemic respiratory failure, showed no significant improvement in 60-day survival.[19] As a result, current guidelines recommend dexamethasone 6 mg daily as the preferred dose for hospitalized COVID-19 patients requiring supplemental oxygen.

Beyond dexamethasone, other corticosteroids like hydrocortisone and methylprednisolone have been explored in COVID-19 treatment trials. However, many of these studies were stopped early due to low enrollment after the promising results of the RECOVERY trial with dexamethasone. This limited data creates weak evidence for using hydrocortisone or methylprednisolone compared to dexamethasone as a standard treatment. The REMAP-CAP trial enrolled critically ill COVID-19 patients requiring intensive care support. This study suggests a potential benefit for hydrocortisone, either in a fixed 7-day dose or shock-dependent regimen, in improving organ-support-free days within 21 days.[20]

Current guidelines recommend dexamethasone 6 mg daily for 7–10 days as the standard corticosteroid therapy for hospitalized COVID-19 patients requiring oxygen support. This can be administered orally or intravenously. If dexamethasone is unavailable, alternative options like prednisone (40 mg daily), methylprednisolone (32 mg daily), or hydrocortisone (160 mg daily) can be considered based on their equivalent anti-inflammatory potency. These doses are derived from dexamethasone's superior potency compared to other options (6.25x prednisolone, 5x methylprednisolone, 25x hydrocortisone).[21,22]

Combining systemic corticosteroids with specific immunomodulators like tocilizumab (IL-6 inhibitor) or baricitinib (Janus kinase inhibitor) can benefit hospitalized COVID-19 patients with early critical illness and systemic inflammation. However, close monitoring is crucial due to potential adverse effects. Steroid use increases the risk of hyperglycemia, infections (including opportunistic fungal infections like mucormycosis and aspergillosis, and reactivation of latent infections like tuberculosis, hepatitis B, herpesviruses, and strongyloidiasis), psychiatric issues and avascular necrosis. Additionally, combining corticosteroids with other immunosuppressants like tocilizumab or baricitinib further elevates the risk of secondary infections, with cases of disseminated strongyloidiasis reported in COVID-19 patients receiving this combination therapy.[23]

Conclusion

In conclusion, corticosteroids, particularly dexamethasone at 6 mg daily, have become a mainstay treatment for hospitalized COVID-19 patients requiring supplemental oxygen. This medication works by dampening the excessive inflammatory response that can lead to lung damage. While other corticosteroids like hydrocortisone show promise, more research is needed to determine their definitive role compared to dexamethasone. The use of corticosteroids should be balanced against potential side effects like infections, hyperglycemia, and avascular necrosis. In severe cases, combining corticosteroids with specific immunomodulators may offer additional benefits, but close monitoring is necessary due to the increased risk of serious infections.

CORTICOSTEROIDS IN ALLERGIC BRONCHOPULMONARY ASPERGILLOSIS

ABPA emerges from an exaggerated immune response to *Aspergillus fumigatus* in genetically predisposed individuals with asthma or cystic fibrosis.[24] Trapped fungal conidia in airway mucus germinate into hyphae, releasing antigens that trigger IgE-mediated hypersensitivity. This inflammatory cascade culminates in bronchial inflammation, bronchospasm, and progressive airway destruction, defining the clinical picture of ABPA.[25]

ABPA management hinges on a dual strategy thus, controlling immunologic hypersensitivity to *Aspergillus fumigatus* and diminishing airway fungal burden, as uncontrolled inflammation can exacerbate colonization and vice versa. Systemic corticosteroids control the inflammatory cascade, while antifungal medication, primarily itraconazole, reduces airway fungal burden and prevents future exacerbations. Despite demonstrably beneficial effects, the optimal dosing schedule for prednisolone in ABPA remains undefined. A widely employed regimen, as outlined by Greenberger (2002), involves an initial daily dose of prednisolone 0.5 mg/kg for 2 weeks, followed by 0.5 mg/kg every other day for 6–8 weeks, with subsequent tapering by 5–10 mg every 2 weeks until complete discontinuation at 3 months.[26] To achieve sustained disease control and minimize the risk of relapse, some patients may need a low-maintenance corticosteroid regimen. Agarwal et al proposed a high-dose regimen starting with prednisolone 0.75 mg/kg/day for 6 weeks, followed by 0.5 mg/kg/day for another 6 weeks, then transitioning to a maintenance dose of 5 mg every 6 weeks for a total duration of 6–12 months.[27,28] Resolution of radiographic infiltrates and normalization of peripheral blood eosinophil counts for 6 months after cessation of oral corticosteroids signify ABPA remission.

Total serum IgE serves as a crucial biomarker for both disease activity assessment and treatment efficacy monitoring in ABPA. Total serum IgE levels are monitored every 6–8 weeks after oral steroid initiation and continued for a year to capture the lowest level as the patient-specific baseline. While normalization may not always be attainable, a 35–50% reduction in total serum IgE generally signifies symptomatic and radiological improvement, highlighting the multifaceted nature of ABPA management. Sequential imaging with chest X-ray or HRCT of the chest is recommended after 4–8 weeks of steroid therapy to assess the resolution of pulmonary infiltrates. Furthermore, serial spirometry proves valuable in monitoring the evolution of lung function throughout the treatment course.[29]

Intravenous pulse methylprednisolone therapy, administered at 10–20 mg/kg/day for three consecutive days with monthly repetition, has emerged as a treatment option for patients experiencing adverse effects from daily steroids or exhibiting resistance to oral therapy.[30] In a recent study, ABPA-S patients treated with formoterol/budesonide (24–1600 µg/day) for 6 months experienced symptomatic deterioration and elevation of total serum IgE levels. These observations add to existing evidence suggesting that inhaled corticosteroids are not a standalone therapy for ABPA.[31]

Antifungal agents play a complementary role in ABPA management by reducing the fungal burden and antigen load, thereby mitigating the inflammatory response. Itraconazole remains the most prevalent antifungal choice, particularly in steroid-resistant cases or for minimizing reliance on high-dose steroids. In adults, the recommended regimen involves 200 mg twice daily for 4–6 months, followed by a gradual taper over another 4–6 months.[32]

Guideline Recommendations for Treatment of ABPA

The ISHAM-ABPA working group recently published revised clinical practice guidelines for diagnosing, classifying, and treating allergic bronchopulmonary aspergillosis/mycoses (Agarwal et al, 2024). These guidelines are being revised to incorporate recent advancements in diagnostic tests like serum A. fumigatus-specific IgG detection and minimal diagnostic level for serum total IgE. Additionally, new treatment strategies based on recent RCTs are being incorporated into the guidelines.[33]

Systemic glucocorticoids, particularly prednisolone, remain the cornerstone of treatment for acute ABPA. While a randomized trial showed similar effectiveness between low and high prednisolone doses in controlling exacerbations, the lower dose resulted in fewer side effects but potentially slower initial response. Therefore, several centers use doses intermediate between the low and high doses (prednisolone 0.5 mg/kg/day, 0.25 mg/kg/day, and 0.125 mg/kg/day for four weeks each, then tapered by 5 mg every two weeks till discontinuation). The DECG recommended using a 4-month course of low-to-moderate dose oral prednisolone (0.5 mg/kg/day for 2–4 weeks, tapered and completed over four months) for acute ABPA.[33]

Initiating Treatment for Newly Diagnosed ABPA

Treatment of newly diagnosed ABPA prioritizes a measured approach based on disease severity. Asymptomatic patients with ABPA do not require systemic therapy. For patients with ABPA-S, treatment with systemic agents is only indicated if they experience poor asthma control or recurrent exacerbations despite optimized asthma therapy. Initial therapy for acute ABPA typically involves a low-to-moderate dose of oral prednisolone (0.5 mg/kg/day for 2–4 weeks) tapered over four months.[33] Oral itraconazole for four months serves as an alternative for patients, where systemic glucocorticoids are contraindicated (Fig. 8.1). Notably, the combination of itraconazole

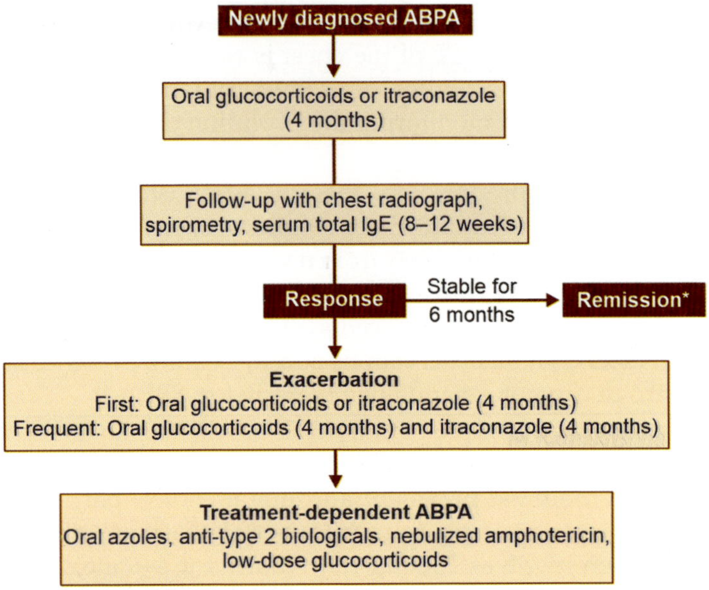

Fig. 8.1: Stage-wise management of patients with ABPA/M[33]

and glucocorticoids is not recommended as first-line therapy, although a brief course of glucocorticoids (<2 weeks) may be used alongside itraconazole initially. While voriconazole, posaconazole, and isavuconazole hold promise, they are reserved for situations with contraindications to systemic glucocorticoids and intolerance, treatment failure, or resistance to itraconazole. High-dose inhaled corticosteroids (ICS) and biological agents are not considered first-line therapies for acute ABPA.

Treatment of ABPA Exacerbation

Management of acute ABPA exacerbations follows a similar approach as initial treatment for newly diagnosed ABPA. However, for recurrent ABPA exacerbations (defined as two or more episodes within the past 1–2 years), a combination of oral prednisolone and itraconazole is recommended.[33] Notably, the use of biological agents and nebulized amphotericin B is not endorsed for treating acute ABPA exacerbations.

Management of Treatment-dependent ABPA

For treatment-dependent ABPA management options include long-term itraconazole, nebulized amphotericin B, and biologics.[33] Continuous low-dose glucocorticosteroids should be considered the least preferred option in this setting.

Management of ABPA in Remission

In remission (stable disease) from ABPA, management focuses on controlling underlying asthma and bronchiectasis with established therapies like inhaled corticosteroids, bronchodilators, antibiotics, and nebulized saline. Additionally, regular monitoring with clinical reviews, serum IgE, and lung function tests (every 3–6 months initially, then every 6–12 months) is crucial.[33] For patients achieving remission on antifungal azoles or biologics, periodic evaluations are recommended to assess the ongoing need for these medications.

Management of Extensive Bronchiectasis and Advanced ABPA

In managing extensive bronchiectasis and advanced ABPA, established guidelines from other pulmonary disorders (chronic obstructive lung disease, ILD, and bronchiectasis) can be applied for long-term oxygen therapy, vaccination strategies, and lung transplantation evaluation.

Treatment during Special Conditions

Management considerations for ABPA vary based on patient characteristics. In pregnancy, systemic glucocorticoids at non-pregnant dosages remain the mainstay for acute or treatment-dependent ABPA, while biological agents and oral azoles are contraindicated due to potential teratogenicity. For cystic fibrosis (CF)-ABPA, the diagnostic and treatment approaches largely mirror those for ABPA in asthmatics, with initial preference for glucocorticoids or azoles. Monthly intravenous methylprednisolone, alone or combined with azoles, may be used to minimize toxicity associated with daily oral steroids in CF patients. Glucocorticoid–azole combinations are becoming increasingly common for CF-ABPA.[33] Pediatric ABPA presents unique challenges, with concerns regarding growth suppression from systemic corticosteroids and variable azole absorption due to immature CYP450 enzymes. Randomized controlled trials for ABPA treatment in children are lacking. While systemic steroids and oral itraconazole are considered for acute ABPA in children as in adults, further research is needed to address the specific therapeutic issues in this population. Omalizumab and mepolizumab are options for children aged 6 years and older, with other biologics potentially suitable for those above 12 years.

Conclusion

Systemic glucocorticoids, particularly prednisolone, remain the cornerstone of treatment for acute ABPA. While both high and low-dose regimens can control exacerbations, lower doses offer the benefit of fewer side effects. To address the potential for slower initial response with lower doses, many centers utilize intermediate tapering regimens. While glucocorticoids are crucial for initial control, they are not a long-term solution for all patients. The emergence of treatment-dependent ABPA necessitates alternative or adjunctive therapies like antifungal medications (itraconazole, nebulized amphotericin B) or biologics. The management of ABPA extends beyond acute episodes. During remission, controlling underlying conditions like asthma and bronchiectasis is essential. Regular monitoring and periodic assessments are crucial for all patients, particularly those on long-term antifungals or biologics.

In conclusion, while steroids remain a vital tool in the ABPA treatment arsenal, the landscape is evolving. Individualized treatment plans that consider disease severity, risk factors, and response to therapy are key to achieving optimal outcomes for patients with ABPA.

STEROIDS IN *PNEUMOCYSTIS JIROVECII*

Pneumocystis jirovecii pneumonia (PCP), previously called *Pneumocystis carinii* pneumonia, is a frequent and potentially life-threatening opportunistic pulmonary infection in patients living with HIV (PLHIV). Approximately 90% of PCP cases occur in individuals with CD4 T lymphocyte counts below 200 cells/mm^3. Typically, PCP presents with a subacute onset of progressive dyspnea, fever, non-productive cough, and chest discomfort, which can worsen significantly within days to weeks. Tachypnea, tachycardia, and diffuse crackles are frequently observed on clinical examination.

Hypoxemia is the hallmark feature of PCP, with severity ranging from mild (PaO_2 70–79 mm Hg) to moderate (PaO_2 60–69 mm Hg) and severe (PaO_2 <60 mm Hg). Chest radiograph typically reveals diffuse, bilateral, symmetrical interstitial infiltrates with a characteristic "ground-glass" appearance. Definitive diagnosis relies on demonstrating the organism, *Pneumocystis jirovecii*, in bronchoalveolar lavage (BAL) specimens. The preferred oral regimen for mild–moderate PCP is TMP-SMX (160 mg/800 mg), two tablets three times daily for 21 days. In moderate–severe cases, intravenous TMP-SMX (TMP 15–20 mg and SMX 75–100 mg/kg/day) every 6 or 8 hours for 21 days is preferred. Alternative therapies like atovaquone or dapsone may be considered for TMP-SMX intolerant patients. Individualized dosing adjustments based on patient factors are recommended.

Adjuvant Steroids in PCP

In patients with *Pneumocystis jirovecii* pneumonia (PCP) exhibiting severe hypoxemia (PaO_2 <70 mm Hg on room air or A-aDO_2 gradient >35 mm Hg), adjunctive corticosteroid therapy with prednisone is recommended to improve oxygenation and potentially reduce mortality. Early initiation, ideally within 72 hours of starting PCP-specific antimicrobials, is crucial for optimal benefit. A standard 21-day oral regimen in adults involves 40 mg twice daily for the first five days, followed by 40 mg once daily for days six to ten and 20 mg once daily for days 11 to 21. For children with severe PCP, a similar tapering schedule is suggested, with 1 mg/kg twice daily for days one to five, 1 mg/kg once daily for days six to ten, and 0.5 mg/kg once daily for days 11 to 21. Ewald et al investigated the potential benefits of adjunctive corticosteroids in improving overall survival and reducing mechanical ventilation requirements among HIV-infected patients with PCP experiencing severe hypoxemia (PaO_2 <70 mm Hg or alveolar-arterial gradient >35 mm Hg on room air)[34] (Table 8.1).

Table 8.1: Prednisolone dosing for PCP management

Age group	*Days 1–5*	*Days 6–10*	*Days 11–21*
Adults	40 mg twice daily	40 mg once daily	20 mg once daily
Children (severe PCP)	1 mg/kg twice daily	1 mg/kg once daily	0.5 mg/kg once daily

STEROIDS IN IMMUNE RECONSTITUTION INFLAMMATORY SYNDROME (IRIS)

IRIS can develop in 10–30% of HIV-infected individuals soon after initiating antiretroviral therapy (ART), typically within the first 4–8 weeks. Chronic HIV infection suppresses CD4 T-lymphocytes, impairing the body's usual response to infections. While ART effectively repairs these immune defects and elevates CD4 counts, this rapid restoration can trigger a disproportionate inflammatory reaction. This manifests as non-specific symptoms like fever, lymph node enlargement, and, in some cases, a paradoxical worsening of pre-existing infections or non-infective conditions. Tuberculosis and cryptococcosis represent the most severe and life-threatening forms of paradoxical IRIS due to their potential for rapid reactivation with immune rebound.

IRIS is generally a self-limiting condition, and ART interruption is rarely indicated. The mild form of IRIS with ongoing ART needs observation. Antimicrobial therapy is required for ongoing infections. Short-course corticosteroids or NSAIDs may mitigate inflammatory symptoms, promoting symptomatic relief. Prednisolone dosing may be employed in a stepwise manner, starting at 1.5 mg/kg orally for 2 weeks, followed by 0.75 mg/ kg orally for 2 weeks, and then gradual tapering based on individual response.[35,36] Temporary ART cessation should be considered only in exceptional cases of potentially life-threatening IRIS, such as severe TB-IRIS or cryptococcal meningitis.

REFERENCES

1. World Health Organization. Global health estimates: life expectancy and leading causes of death and disability. Accessed December 18, 2020. https://www.who.int/data/gho/data/themes/mortality-and-global-health-estimates.
2. Harris LK, Crannage AJ. Corticosteroids in Community-Acquired Pneumonia: A Review of Current Literature. Journal of Pharmacy Technology. 2021;37(3):152–60. doi:10.1177/8755122521995587.
3. Stern A, Skalsky K, Avni T, Carrara E, Leibovici L, Paul M. Corticosteroids for pneumonia. Cochrane Database Syst Rev. 2017;(12):CD007720. doi: 10.1002/14651858.CD007720.pub3.
4. Briel M, Spoorenberg SMC, Snijders D, et al. Corticosteroids in patients hospitalized with community-acquired pneumonia: systematic review and individual patient data meta-analysis. Clin Infect Dis. 2018;66:346–354. doi: 10.1093/cid/cix801.
5. Confalonieri M, Urbino R, Potena A, Piattella M, Parigi P, Puccio G, Della Porta R, Giorgio C, Blasi F, Umberger R, Meduri GU. Hydrocortisone infusion for severe community-acquired pneumonia: a preliminary randomized study. Am J Respir Crit Care Med. 2005 Feb 1;171(3):242–8. doi: 10.1164/rccm.200406-808OC. Epub 2004 Nov 19. PMID: 15557131.
6. Meduri GU, Shih M-C, Bridges L, Martin TJ, El-Solh A, Seam N, et al. Low-dose methylprednisolone treatment in critically ill patients with severe community-acquired pneumonia. Intensive Care Med 2022;48:1009–23. http:// dx.doi.org/10.1007/s00134-022-06684-3.
7. Dequin P-F, Meziani F, Quenot J-P, Kamel T, Ricard J-D, Badie J, et al. Hydrocortisone in severe community-acquired pneumonia. N Engl J Med 2023. http://dx.doi.org/10.1056/NEJMoa2215145. NEJMoa2215145.
8. Mandell LA, Wunderink RG, Anzueto A, et al. Infectious Diseases Society of America/American Thoracic Society consensus guidelines on the management of community-acquired pneumonia in adults. Clin Infect Dis. 2007;44(suppl 2): S27-S72. doi: 10.1086/511159.
9. Metlay JP, Waterer GW, Long AC, et al. Diagnosis and treatment of adults with community-acquired pneumonia. An official clinical practice guideline of the American Thoracic Society and Infectious Diseases Society of America. Am J Respir Crit Care Med. 2019;200:e45-e67. doi: 10.1164/rccm.201908-1581ST.
10. Boyles TH, Brink A, Calligaro GL, Cohen C, Dheda K, Maartens G, Richards GA, van Zyl Smit R, Smith C, Wasserman S, Whitelaw AC, Feldman C; South African Thoracic Society; Federation of Infectious Diseases Societies of Southern Africa. South African guideline for the management of community-acquired pneumonia in adults. J Thorac Dis. 2017 Jun;9(6):1469–1502. doi: 10.21037/jtd.2017.05.31. Erratum in: J Thorac Dis. 2018 Aug;10(8): E673-E675. PMID: 28740661; PMCID: PMC5506119.
11. Martin-Loeches I, Torres A, Nagavci B, et al. ERS/ESICM/ESCMID/ALAT guidelines for the management of severe community-acquired pneumonia. Eur Respir J 2023;61:2200735[DOI: 10.1183/13993003.00735-2022].
12. Martin-Loeches I, Lisboa T, Rhodes A, et al. Use of early corticosteroid therapy on ICU admission in patients affected by severe pandemic (H1N1) v influenza A infection. Intensive Care Med 2011; 37: 272–83. doi:10.1007/s00134-010-2078-z.

13. Brun-Buisson C, Richard JC, Mercat A, Thiebaut AC, Brochard L. Early corticosteroids in severe influenza A/H1N1 pneumonia and acute respiratory distress syndrome. *American Journal of Respiratory and Critical Care Medicine* 2011;183:1200–1206, https://doi.org/10.1164/rccm.201101-0135OC.
14. Metlay JP, Waterer GW, Long AC, et al. Diagnosis and treatment of adults with community-acquired pneumonia. An official clinical practice guideline of the American Thoracic Society and Infectious Diseases Society of America. *Am J Respir Crit Care Med.* 2019;200:e45–67. doi: 10.1164/rccm.201908-1581ST.
15. Ni YN, Chen G, Sun J, et al. The effect of corticosteroids on mortality of patients with influenza pneumonia: a systematic review and meta-analysis. Crit Care 2019;23:99. doi:10.1186/s13054-019-2395-8.
16. Yang J-W, Yang L, Luo R-G, et al. Corticosteroid administration for viral pneumonia: COVID-19 and beyond. Clin Microbiol Infect 2020;26:1171–77. doi:10.1016/j.cmi.2020.06.02.
17. RECOVERY Collaborative Group. Dexamethasone in hospitalized patients with COVID-19. *N Engl J Med.* 2021;384(8):693–704. Available at: https://www.ncbi.nlm.nih.gov/pubmed/32678530.
18. COVID STEROID 2 Trial Group. Effect of 12 mg vs 6 mg of dexamethasone on the number of days alive without life support in adults with COVID-19 and severe hypoxemia: the COVID STEROID 2 randomized trial. JAMA. 2021;326(18):1807–17. Available at: https://www.ncbi.nlm.nih.gov/pubmed/34673895.
19. Bouadma L, Mekontso-Dessap A, Burdet C, et al. High-dose dexamethasone and oxygen support strategies in intensive care unit patients with severe COVID-19 acute hypoxemic respiratory failure: the COVIDICUS randomized clinical trial. JAMA Intern Med. 2022;182(9):906–916. Available at: https://www.ncbi.nlm.nih.gov/pubmed/35788622.
20. REMAP-CAP Investigators. Interleukin-6 receptor antagonists in critically ill patients with COVID-19. N Engl J Med. 2021;384(16):1491–1502. Available at: https://www.ncbi.nlm.nih.gov/pubmed/33631065.
21. Dequin PF, Heming N, Meziani F, et al. Effect of hydrocortisone on 21-day mortality or respiratory support among critically ill patients with COVID-19: a randomized clinical trial. JAMA. 2020;324(13):1298–1306. Available at: https://www.ncbi.nlm.nih.gov/pubmed/32876689.
22. Czock D, Keller F, Rasche FM, Häussler U. Pharmacokinetics and pharmacodynamics of systemically administered glucocorticoids. Clin Pharmacokinet. 2005;44(1):61–98. Available at: https://www.ncbi.nlm.nih.gov/pubmed/15634032.
23. Lier AJ, Tuan JJ, Davis MW, et al. Case report: disseminated strongyloidiasis in a patient with COVID-19. AmJ Trop Med Hyg. 2020;103(4):1590–92. Available at: https://www.ncbi.nlm.nih.gov/pubmed/32830642.
24. Janahi IA, Rehman A, Al-Naimi AR. Allergic bronchopulmonary aspergillosis in patients with cystic fibrosis. Annals of Thoracic Medicine. 2017;12(2):74.
25. Knutsen AP, Bush RK, Demain JG, Denning DW, Dixit A, Fairs A, et al. Fungi and allergic lower respiratory tract diseases. *J Allergy Clin Immunol* 2012;129:280–91.
26. Greenberger PA. Allergic bronchopulmonary aspergillosis. *J Allergy Clin Immunol.* 2002;110:685–92.
27. Agarwal R. Allergic bronchopulmonary aspergillosis. Chest. 2009;135:805–26.
28. Agarwal R, Gupta D, Agarwal AN, et al. Allergic bronchopulmonary aspergillosis: lessons from 126 patients attending chest clinic in North India. Chest. 2006;130:442–48.
29. Mahdavinia M, Grammer LC. Management of allergic bronchopulmonary aspergillosis: a review and update. Ther Adv Respir Dis. 2012;6(3):173–87.
30. Singh Sehgal I, Agarwal R. Pulse methylprednisolone in allergic bronchopulmonary aspergillosis exacerbations. Eur Respir Rev. 2014;23:149–52.
31. Agarwal R, Khan A, Aggarwal AN, Saikia B, Gupta D, Chakrabarti A. Role of inhaled corticosteroids in the management of serological allergic bronchopulmonary aspergillosis (ABPA) Intern Med. 2011;50:855–60.

32. Agarwal R. What is the current place of azoles in allergic bronchopulmonary aspergillosis and severe asthma with fungal sensitization? Expert Rev Respir Med. 2012;6:363–71.
33. Revised clinical practice guidelines for diagnosing, classifying, and treating allergic bronchopulmonary aspergillosis/mycoses: a Delphi statement from the ISHAM-ABPA working group Ritesh Agarwal, Inderpaul Singh Sehgal, Valliappan Muthu, David W Denning, Arunaloke Chakrabarti, Kathirvel Soundappan, Mandeep Garg, Shivaprakash M Rudramurthy, Sahajal Dhooria, Darius Armstrong-James, Koichiro Asano, Jean-Pierre Gangneux, Sanjay H Chotirmall, Helmut JF Salzer, James D Chalmers, Cendrine Godet, Marcus Joest, Iain Page, Parameswaran Nair, p Arjun, Raja Dhar, Kana Ram Jat, Geethu Joe, Uma Maheswari Krishnaswamy, Joseph L Mathew, Venkata Nagarjuna Maturu, Anant Mohan, Alok Nath, Dharmesh Patel, Jayanthi Savio, Puneet Saxena, Rajeev Soman, Balamugesh Thangakunam, Caroline G Baxter, Felix Bongomin, William J Calhoun, Oliver A Cornely, Jo A Douglass, Chris Kosmidis, Jacques F Meis, Richard Moss, Alessandro C Pasqualotto, Danila Seidel, Rosanne Sprute, Kuruswamy Thurai Prasad, Ashutosh N Aggarwal. *European Respiratory Journal Jan* 2024, 2400061; DOI: 10.1183/13993003.00061-2024.
34. Ewald H, Raatz H, Boscacci R, Furrer H, Bucher HC, Briel M. Adjunctive corticosteroids for *Pneumocystis jirovecii* pneumonia in patients with HIV infection. Cochrane Database Syst Rev. 2015;4:CD006150.
35. Bell C, Nelson M, Kaye S. A case of immune reconstitution rheumatoid arthritis. *Int J STD AIDS.* 2002;13(8):580–1.
36. Quinn CM, Poplin V, Kasibante J, Yuquimpo K, Gakuru J, Cresswell FV, Bahr NC. Tuberculosis IRIS: Pathogenesis, Presentation, and Management across the Spectrum of Disease. Life (Basel). 2020 Oct 29;10(11):262. doi: 10.3390/life10110262. PMID: 33138069; PMCID: PMC7693460.

Chapter

9

Steroids in Tuberculosis

R Vinod Kumar • Chakrahari Ugandhar Bhattu

INTRODUCTION

The aphorism "Let no man die without a trial of ATT or steroids" highlights the historical dilemma surrounding steroid use in tuberculosis (TB). Steroids are double-edged weapons that have been known from time immemorial. The usage of steroids in any situation needs an analysis of the risks versus benefits accrued in the process.[1] Before the advent of anti-tuberculous chemotherapy, steroids were shown to flare up infections in both animals and humans. Hence, it was suggested that steroids were contraindicated in the presence of tuberculosis.[2] However, later studies have demonstrated beneficial effects in certain situations of tuberculosis infection when steroids have been used with anti-tuberculous therapy.[3] It is seen in tuberculosis that in addition to the overwhelming infection, the inflammatory reaction to *Mycobacterium tuberculosis* can result in significant tissue damage. Resultant healing by fibrosis can also damage multiple organ systems. Steroids have been used in the management of cases of Tuberculosis to suppress the unwanted inflammatory events arising in response to infection with *Mycobacterium tuberculosis*. The fear stems from the immunosuppressive effect of steroids, which may worsen the outcome of tuberculosis if used routinely in the management of tuberculosis.[4]

CURRENT SCENARIOS WHERE STEROIDS ARE USED IN TUBERCULOSIS

A specific indication for the use of steroids is adrenocortical failure caused by tuberculosis. Currently, steroids are being used as adjunctive therapy in TB meningitis, TB pericarditis, and occasionally in pleural tuberculosis, especially in patients with pleurisy manifested as pleuritic chest pain, though the indication in pleural effusion remains debatable. Corticosteroids have been used to support the treatment of severe consequences of TB, such as miliary TB and respiratory insufficiency.

Various studies have used steroids in TB lymphadenitis with promising results.[5,6] It is now being used when new nodes develop, or there is a paradoxical worsening after starting tuberculous chemotherapy due to immune restitution inflammatory syndrome (IRIS) while treating TB lymphadenitis. Similar Jarisch-Herxheimer-like reactions have been observed in the treatment of other forms of tuberculosis, like chorioretinitis, and have been successfully treated with steroids.[7] Steroids may also be required in the management of adverse skin reactions to anti-tuberculous chemotherapy.[8,9] Steroids have also shown beneficial effects in miliary tuberculosis and patients with ARDS.[10]

One definitive indication for steroids in tuberculosis is adrenal insufficiency or Addison's disease. When Thomas Addison first described these cases in 1855, not surprisingly, all were cases of tuberculosis with adrenal involvement. The difficulty in diagnosing adrenal insufficiency stems from its nonspecific and overlapping symptoms with tuberculosis, including fatigue, weakness, loss of weight, and appetite. A clue to the diagnosis could be low blood pressure, and confirmation could be by detection of adrenal enlargement in imaging and measurement of cortisol levels. Few cases have demonstrated the mycobacteria and granulomatous inflammation in adrenal biopsy.[11,12]

The 2020 WHO guidelines recommend corticosteroids primarily for two extrapulmonary TB scenarios:

1. **Tuberculous meningitis:** Adjuvant therapy with dexamethasone/prednisolone (6–8 weeks) alongside anti-tuberculous treatment (ATT) reduces mortality, disability, and relapse, with benefits increasing for severe cases. Notably, steroid-treated patients experience fewer adverse events like severe hepatitis.
2. **Tuberculous pericarditis:** Corticosteroids are considered due to potential benefits, including reduced mortality, constrictive pericarditis risk, and improved treatment adherence. These recommendations mainly apply to non-MDR/RR-TB but may extend to MDR/RR-TB patients on effective treatment. However, due to their immunosuppressive nature, they should be strictly limited to clear indications with established adequate ATT adherence, as inadequate regimens can worsen outcomes. Oral corticosteroids are standard, but injectables may be preferred initially for faster response.

MECHANISM OF ACTION OF CORTICOSTEROIDS IN TB

Despite well-understood molecular and cellular actions, the specific roles of corticosteroids in diverse diseases, including TB, remain under investigation. Corticosteroids dampen inflammation through multiple pathways: binding DNA elements (GREs) to regulate gene expression, blocking key transcription factors (NF-κB), and modulating signaling cascades. While the exact mechanism remains elusive, their benefits likely stem from suppressing proinflammatory cytokines like TNF-α, reducing neutrophil influx, and reversing vascular permeability, ultimately alleviating tissue damage and improving function in severe TB forms like meningitis or pericarditis. However, it is crucial to acknowledge the incomplete understanding of their exact targets and the potential downsides of immunosuppression, necessitating their cautious use within a comprehensive TB treatment plan.

STEROID USAGE IN SPECIFIC FORMS OF TUBERCULOSIS

Pulmonary Tuberculosis

The role of corticosteroids in pulmonary tuberculosis, which accounts for more than 80% of tuberculosis, remains a matter of debate. Studies in the 1950s and 60s[13] demonstrated a quicker reduction of fever, quicker clinical recovery, quicker correction of anaemia, and rapid normalization of radiological findings when steroids were added to the chemotherapy, especially in the fulminant form of tuberculosis. However, subsequent studies did not show any benefits at the end of 6 months, especially concerning pulmonary function.[14] However, there is a fear of flare-ups and worsening of pulmonary tuberculosis due to the immunosuppressive effects of steroids. Also, the high prevalence of both diabetes mellitus and HIV in the Indian scenario precludes its widespread use in high-burden situations.

In childhood tuberculosis[15] has been tried, especially in endobronchial TB, but benefits were not seen at the end of treatment. Random case reports as the one published by the author of an 18-year-old girl with total lung collapse due to endobronchial TB who recovered with a course of anti-TB therapy with steroids, do exist.[16]

Currently, steroids are used mainly in tuberculosis with respiratory failure like miliary tuberculosis and in tuberculous ARDS in which there is a demonstrable mortality reduction benefit.[10] Steroids can also be used in situations like documented adrenal insufficiency, the presence of pericardial effusion, and for managing severe drug rashes if they develop during treatment with anti-tuberculous chemotherapy.

As mentioned earlier, a risk-benefit analysis should be done before administering steroids as an adjunct to tuberculous therapy in pulmonary tuberculosis patients.

Pleural Tuberculosis

Pleural tuberculosis can develop in up to 30% of patients with tuberculosis. It results from either a rupture of subpleural tuberculous focus into the pleural space or due to an immunological reaction in primary infection, especially in young adults. The rationale for corticosteroid use in pleural TB rests on its ability to dampen the exuberant type IV hypersensitivity response triggered by released mycobacterial antigens. The main intent of treatment is to prevent the development of pleural adhesions, which can compromise respiratory function in the future, and also to prevent the development of parenchymal tuberculosis in the future.

Several studies in the past have attempted to study the effects of the addition of steroids to standard therapy, both non-randomized and randomized trials, but the evidence generated has not been statistically significant to recommend the routine use of steroids in all cases of pleural effusions.[4] Clinically, we do use steroids, especially in cases where continue to have pleuritic pain despite the use of ATT, where steroids have a mitigating effect on the pain by reducing the pleural inflammation, but further studies are needed to justify the use of steroids in such a scenario.

The efficacy of adjunctive corticosteroids in treating tuberculous pleural effusion remains a topic of debate. A recent Cochrane meta-analysis by Ryan et al encompassing 6 trials with 590 participants, investigated their potential benefits. The analysis suggested that corticosteroids may expedite pleural effusion resolution and minimize the risk of chronic pleural thickening and adhesions. However, data regarding their impact on post-treatment respiratory function remains inconclusive. Notably, corticosteroid use carries an increased risk of adverse events necessitating treatment discontinuation. Epigastric pain, hypertension, and hyperglycemia are frequently reported side effects. Current programmatic guidelines recommend treating pleural effusions only with ATT.[17,18]

Tuberculous Meningitis

If at all, there appears to be some consensus on the usage of steroids in TB, it is in TB meningitis. Current national and WHO guidelines recommend the use of adjuvant steroids in the treatment of TB meningitis, given its high mortality and potential for severe neurological deficits in survivors. However, it is also recommended to review the use after a month of therapy and taper the dose as soon as it is deemed safe. Tuberculous meningitis occurs when a subependymal focus ruptures into the subarachnoid space and involves meningitis, which is the commonest part of the CNS to be involved in the infection. Encephalitis, arteritis, and vasculitis have also been documented. Patients present with various neurological involvement, including cranial nerve palsies and stroke, due to inflammation involvement of the circle of Willis and the basal meninges.

While controlled and uncontrolled trials have not consistently shown a positive response to steroid therapy for tuberculous meningitis (TBM), their ability to reduce early cerebral edema and potentially decrease mortality in specific patient groups remains a compelling argument for their use. Despite meta-analyses failing to demonstrate long-term benefits in preventing neurological complications, the high mortality and neurological sequelae associated with TBM warrant continued consideration of steroids in specific patient subsets. Current recommendations suggest their use for patients with TBM classified as at least grade II or III on the British Research Council scale (**Stage I:** Mild, no altered consciousness or focal neurological signs; **Stage II:** Moderately advanced, impaired consciousness but not comatose with moderate deficits; **Stage III:** Comatose with multiple deficits including cranial nerve palsies and bilateral signs). The rationale lies in potentially mitigating the detrimental effects of the inflammatory response in these severe cases, even if long-term outcomes have not been universally confirmed. Despite conflicting evidence, Kameswara Prasad et al demonstrated a potential mortality benefit with corticosteroid use in TB meningitis (32% vs 41% mortality).[18]

Steroids in HIV-negative patients can be recommended for at least 4 weeks, but in HIV-positive patients, steroids may be used after ruling out opportunistic infections, e.g. cryptococcal meningitis and cerebral toxoplasmosis—as these are associated with increased mortality with the use of steroids. The preferred regimen entails administering intravenous dexamethasone at 0.4 mg/kg/day divided into 3–4 doses during hospitalization. If intravenous administration is not feasible, switch to oral dexamethasone at 0.4 mg/kg/day in divided doses or prednisone at 1 mg/kg/day in a single morning dose. Upon discharge, initiate a tapering regimen of oral corticosteroids for a total duration of 8–12 weeks (e.g. IV dexamethasone 0.4 mg/kg × 2 weeks → 0.3 mg/kg × 1 week → 0.2 mg/kg × 1 week → followed by 4 mg/day × 1 week × 3 mg/day × 1 week → 2 mg/day × 1 week → 1 mg/day × 1 week).[18]

Tuberculous Pericarditis

Current guidelines favor the use of steroids in patients with tuberculous pericarditis since various trials have shown mortality benefits and some reduction in the development of constrictive pericarditis is started early on in the course of the illness, but the evidence remains equivocal, leaving it to the clinician to use his judicious judgement on a case to case basis.[3,4] Tuberculous pericarditis has been documented in up to 1% of patients with tuberculosis and progresses through three phases—exudative, exude-constrictive, and constrictive phases. If steroids are started early on in the exudative phase, it might prevent the development of the dreaded constrictive pericarditis, which is associated with much morbidity and mortality.

Corticosteroids play a key role in managing TB pericarditis, particularly in specific scenarios characterized by significant inflammatory activity. These include large pericardial effusions, prominent pleocytosis (inflammatory cells in pericardial fluid), effusions with elevated inflammatory markers, and early pericardial constriction.[18] The recommended dosing regimen typically involves prednisone administered at 1 mg/kg daily for 4 weeks, followed by a gradual taper to 0.5 mg/kg daily for another 4 weeks before further gradual tapering over 2–4 weeks. Alternatively, an equivalent prednisolone regimen can be employed, starting with 60 mg/day for 4 weeks, then 30 mg/day for 4 weeks, tapered to 15 mg/day for 2 weeks, followed by 5 mg/day for 1 week, and stop. The total duration of systemic steroids is 11 weeks, depending on the regimen that may be used.[18] The specific approach may vary based on individual patient factors and response to therapy. Regardless of the chosen regimen, close monitoring for potential side effects and judicious tapering remain crucial during corticosteroid therapy for TB pericarditis.

Intraocular TB

For paramacular and optic nerve head tuberculosis, the mainstay therapy combines anti-tuberculous drugs (ATT) with systemic corticosteroids. Oral prednisolone at 1 mg/kg/day is initiated, followed by a gradual taper based on individual clinical response. In cases of severe anterior chamber inflammation, topical steroid eye drops may be employed as an adjunct therapy.[18]

Endobronchial Tuberculosis (EBTB)

Endobronchial tuberculosis (EBTB), also known as tracheobronchial TB, is a distinct form of pulmonary tuberculosis characterized by the direct infection of the tracheobronchial tree with *Mycobacterium tuberculosis*, confirmed by both microbiological and histopathological evidence. While Richard Morton, an English physician, first described tracheobronchial TB in 1698, its diagnosis remains challenging due to the frequent absence of telltale signs on chest X-rays, often leading to delayed treatment. To overcome this hurdle, advanced investigations like computed tomography (CT) scanning and bronchoscopy are crucial for definitive diagnosis and evaluation of bronchial lesions, such as stenosis or obstruction. The clinical spectrum of EBTB is diverse, with active disease typically presenting with cough, hemoptysis, sputum production, wheezing, chest pain, and fever. As the disease progresses to a fibrotic stage, dyspnea and persistent wheezing become more prominent. The cornerstone of EBTB management in the active phase lies in eradicating the tubercle bacilli and preventing the development of bronchial stenosis, which can significantly impact lung function.

While corticosteroids hold promise in early EBTB stages, characterized by hypersensitivity, their utility in later fibrotic phases remains uncertain due to potential detrimental effects and lack of conclusive evidence for preventing bronchostenosis in adults. The anti-inflammatory properties of corticosteroids have been explored for their potential to reduce local pressure and inflammation in endobronchial tuberculosis (EBTB).[19,20] Notably, early studies, such as Nemir et al, suggest positive clinical outcomes in children, possibly due to their ability to prevent bronchial compression from inflamed lymph nodes. Park et al found no significant difference in healing rates or lung function between corticosteroid and non-corticosteroid groups in adults, highlighting the importance of early diagnosis and treatment before fibrosis sets in. Notably, they utilized prednisolone at 1 mg/kg for 4–6 weeks in specific presentations (edematous-hyperemic, actively caseating, and tumorous) prone to tracheobronchial stenosis. However, Um et al found no reduction in persistent airway stenosis with higher doses of oral corticosteroids, suggesting their limitations in preventing long-term complications. These conflicting findings underscore the need for further research to define specific scenarios where corticosteroids might be beneficial in EBTB management while balancing potential risks and ensuring optimal long-term outcomes.

Rikimaru's study investigated the potential of local therapy, demonstrating that an aerosol combination of dexamethasone 0.5 mg, streptomycin 100 mg, and naphazoline 0.1 mg administered twice daily alongside conventional oral therapy resulted in faster healing of ulcerative lesions and reduced severity of bronchial stenosis.[21] Submucosal injections of methylprednisolone, for instance, have also shown promising results in resolving EBTB.[22,23] However, the inconsistent evidence across various delivery methods underscores the need for larger, prospective trials before definitively recommending corticosteroids for routine use in adult EBTB patients. In inactive diseases with stenosis, mechanical interventions like surgery or endobronchial procedures are necessary, as steroids and other medications cannot reverse fibrous damage.

CORTICOSTEROIDS IN PEDIATRIC TB

Corticosteroids can play a crucial role in specific scenarios of pediatric TB, but their use requires careful consideration and individualization due to their nuanced role in general management. In critically ill children with hypoxic respiratory distress from miliary TB, they can be lifesaving. Early administration of endobronchial TB might prevent bronchial stenosis by reducing airway inflammation. Extensive organ involvement in disseminated TB offers potential benefits by mitigating inflammation and improving clinical outcomes. Recommended regimens typically involve prednisone (2 mg/kg/day) or dexamethasone (0.6 mg/kg/day) for 4 weeks, followed by a gradual 4-week taper, applicable to both miliary and endobronchial TB. For TB meningitis, prednisone (2 mg/kg/day) with a 4-week taper is advised. Equivalent doses of alternative steroid formulations can be used based on individual needs. Importantly, corticosteroid use in pediatric TB must be individualized, considering specific disease manifestations, severity, and potential risks. Close monitoring for adverse effects and ensuring adherence to anti-tuberculous treatment remain crucial throughout therapy.[24]

STEROIDS IN OTHER SCENARIOS OF TUBERCULOSIS

Multiple anecdotal case reports of usage of steroids in genitourinary TB, choreo uveitis, drug-induced fever, and Poncet's rheumatism have been reported in the literature, but evidence supporting the use in other situations remains debatable at present, and further larger studies are needed to firmly justify the use of steroids in tuberculosis.

Adrenal Gland Insufficiency

In 1855, Addison first described Addison's disease, attributing it to bilateral adrenal gland destruction by tuberculosis (TB) in his patients. While TB remains the most common cause of adrenal insufficiency in developing nations, its declining incidence in the Western world reflects the success of antituberculous chemotherapy. While nonspecific symptoms often delay diagnosis, the life-threatening adrenal crisis can be the initial presentation.

Pathologically, affected adrenal glands typically appear enlarged with extensive caseous necrosis. While the classic granulomatous reaction with numerous epithelioid histiocytes is characteristically observed in extra-adrenal sites of tuberculosis infection, it is notably absent within the adrenal gland. This suggests that the locally high levels of adrenal corticosteroids effectively suppress the host's inflammatory response, contributing to the unique presentation and potential for delayed diagnosis.

Adrenal tuberculosis follows the same treatment approach as other extrapulmonary TB lesions. The mainstay of treatment remains conventional antitubercular therapy, typically involving a standard four-drug regimen. However, the presence of adrenal insufficiency necessitates additional considerations. Lifelong hormone replacement therapy with both glucocorticoids and mineralocorticoids becomes essential. For mineralocorticoid replacement, once-daily fludrocortisone (0.05–0.2 mg) is commonly used. Several options exist for glucocorticoid replacement in adrenal tuberculosis-related insufficiency. Common choices include hydrocortisone (15–25 mg in 2–3 divided doses, with the largest dose in the morning, e.g. 10 mg at waking, 5 mg mid-day, and 2.5 mg late afternoon at 6 pm to mimic the natural cortisol rhythm), prednisone (5 mg orally at bedtime), or dexamethasone (0.75 mg orally at bedtime).[24,26] Children typically receive hydrocortisone at around 8 mg/m^2/day.[27] Monitoring is essential to personalize therapy. Close attention to clinical symptoms and morning plasma ACTH levels helps determine the most effective dosage and regimen for each individual.

Tailoring the specific regimen to individual patient needs and potential drug interactions is crucial. Collaboration with an endocrinologist experienced in managing adrenal insufficiency is highly recommended for optimal patient outcomes.

Lymph Node TB

Peripheral lymph node tuberculosis (PLNTB), most commonly affecting the cervical region, is the leading form of extrapulmonary tuberculosis. Cervical lymph nodes, often referred to as "scrofula," are the primary targets in extrapulmonary tuberculosis, but involvement can extend to supraclavicular, axillary, and inguinal nodes as well. These enlarged lymph nodes (lymphadenopathy) can cause complications like compression of surrounding structures, organs, blood vessels, or even sinus formation.

While multiple studies suggest potential benefits of adding steroids to anti-tuberculosis treatment in various extrapulmonary forms (pleural effusion, pericardial effusion, and mediastinal lymphadenopathy), the safety and efficacy of this approach, specifically for cervical lymphadenopathy, remain largely inconclusive. While controlled trials exist evaluating corticosteroid use in tuberculous lymphadenitis, they predominantly focused on children and specifically targeted mediastinal lymph node involvement, often identified through bronchoscopy or chest X-ray. One notable study by Nemir et al (1965)[24] investigated this approach in 117 children using a blinded, randomized, placebo-controlled design. Serial bronchoscopies were performed by the same investigator, who remained blinded to treatment allocation to assess disease progression.[28] The study reported significant improvement in 67.2% of the prednisone group compared to 45.7% receiving placebo ($p<0.05$). Interestingly, the benefits seemed to be magnified with earlier corticosteroid initiation. An additional study in Indian adults with cervical lymphadenitis revealed similar advantages: faster symptom relief, reduced local complications, and improved lymph node resolution at six months in the prednisolone group compared to the placebo group. These findings suggest the potential benefits of corticosteroids in specific patient populations with tuberculous lymphadenitis, warranting further research to optimize treatment strategies.[29–31]

TUBERCULOSIS-ASSOCIATED IMMUNE RECONSTITUTION INFLAMMATORY SYNDROME

TB-associated immune reconstitution inflammatory syndrome (TB-IRIS) presents in two forms: Unmasking (newly diagnosed TB upon ART initiation) and paradoxical (worsening treated TB after ART). Both share similar mechanisms: a restored immune response against *Mycobacterium tuberculosis* leads to an exaggerated inflammatory reaction. Clinical features encompass fever, respiratory worsening, swollen lymph nodes (with potential abscesses), TB abscesses, and fluid build-up. Central nervous system involvement is particularly severe, and dissemination can occur in severely immunocompromised individuals.

Predictors include low pre-ART CD4 count, high HIV viral load, severe TB, and short interval between TB and ART initiation. Most cases occur within 3 months of starting TB treatment. IRIS is generally a self-limiting condition, and ART interruption is rarely indicated. Mild–moderate TB-IRIS can be managed with supportive care or nonsteroidal anti-inflammatory drugs (though with limited evidence). Severe cases respond well to corticosteroids, as demonstrated by a randomized trial showing symptom improvement without adverse effects. Prednisolone dosing may be employed in a stepwise manner, starting at 1.5 mg/kg orally for 2 weeks, followed by 0.75 mg/kg orally for 2 weeks, and then gradual tapering based on individual response.[32] Stopping either TB therapy or ART is contraindicated.

In conclusion, managing TB-IRIS in HIV/TB co-infection requires careful consideration of individual factors, CD4 count, and potential benefits and risks of early ART initiation. Prednisone co-initiation may offer a promising strategy to reduce TB-IRIS risks, particularly for patients with low CD4 counts starting early ART.[33]

CORTICOSTEROID–ANTITUBERCULAR DRUG INTERACTIONS

The co-administration of corticosteroids with antitubercular drugs necessitates careful attention due to potential interactions affecting their respective therapeutic levels. Prednisolone can decrease isoniazid concentrations through two mechanisms: increased acetylation and enhanced renal clearance. However, this effect is mitigated by the co-administration of rifampicin, a potent inducer of CYP3A4 enzymes that accelerates corticosteroid metabolism and clearance. This interaction is particularly relevant for rapid acetylators, where rifampicin effectively maintains isoniazid levels. Conversely, slow acetylators remain susceptible to reduced isoniazid concentrations even with rifampicin, necessitating closer monitoring.[33] Prednisone can elevate pyrazinamide concentrations within pleural fluid, potentially enhancing its local activity, but does not significantly affect its systemic levels. Remember, attentive monitoring and appropriate dose adjustments are vital when using this drug combination to optimize treatment and minimize adverse effects.

Conclusion

While the role of corticosteroids in tuberculosis (TB) remains a complex balancing act, their potential to mitigate inflammation offers valuable benefits in specific scenarios. In severe forms like miliary TB with hypoxia or disseminated disease, corticosteroids can be lifesaving by reducing inflammation and improving respiratory function. For tuberculous meningitis, they demonstrably decrease mortality and disability risks, particularly when initiated early. In endobronchial TB, corticosteroids may prevent bronchial stenosis and improve airway patency. However, their immunosuppressive nature underscores the need for cautious use, restricted to clearly indicated cases with ongoing effective anti-tuberculous treatment. Ultimately, the decision to employ corticosteroids in TB hinges on a meticulous assessment of disease severity, potential benefits, and individual patient factors, ensuring their judicious integration into the overall treatment plan.

REFERENCES

1. Mandell BF. Balancing the myths of corticosteroid therapy. Clevland clinic journal of medicine 2022; 89(9):480–1.
2. American Trudeau Society. The effect of cortisone and/or corticotropin on tuberculous infection in man. Am Rev Tuberc 1952;66:245–56.
3. A.H. Alzeer, J. M. FitzGerald .Corticosteroids and tuberculosis: risks and use as adjunct therapy. Tubercle and lung diseases 1993;74:6–11.
4. Evans DJ. The use of adjunctive corticosteroids in the treatment of pericardial, pleural and meningeal tuberculosis: Do they improve outcome? Respiratory Medicine 2008;102:793–800.
5. Bunkar ML, Agnihotri SP, Gupta PR, Arya S. Add-on prednisolone in the management of cervical lymph node tuberculosis. Indian J Tuberc. 2016 Apr;63(2):96–99. doi: 10.1016/j.ijtb.2015.05.002. Epub 2016 Jun 4. PMID: 27451818.
6. Sharmin A, Hossain A, Islam N, Sarker ZH, Hossain SS, Khan MA. Outcome of lymph node tuberculosis management with conventional treatment with and without prednisolone. Trop Doct. 2021 Jul;51(3):288–291. doi: 10.1177/0049475520984745. Epub 2021 Jan 10. PMID: 33427091.
7. Cheung CM, Chee SP. Jarisch-Herxheimer reaction: paradoxical worsening of tuberculosis chorioretinitis following initiation of antituberculous therapy. Eye (Lond). 2009 Jun;23(6):1472–3. doi: 10.1038/eye.2008.204. Epub 2008 Jul 4. PMID: 18600241.
8. Sharma RK, Verma GK, Tegta GR, Sood S, Rattan R, Gupta M. Spectrum of Cutaneous Adverse Drug Reactions to Anti-tubercular Drugs and Safe Therapy after Re-challenge: A Retrospective Study. Indian Dermatol Online J. 2020 Mar 9;11(2):177–181. doi: 10.4103/idoj.IDOJ_133_19. PMID: 32477975; PMCID: PMC7247648.
9. Modi, et al. Spectrum of anti tubercular therapy induced cutaneous adverse drug reactions and its management through rechallenge: A prospective study at a Tertiary Care Centre. Indian Journal of Tuberculosis 2022;69(4):470–75.
10. Wakamatsu, et al. Efficacy of steroid pulse therapy for miliary tuberculosis complicated by acute respiratory distress syndrome. *Journal of clinical tuberculosis and mycobacterial diseases* 2022; 29:100341.
11. van Haren Noman S, Visser H, Muller AF, Limonard GJ. Addison's Disease Caused by Tuberculosis: Diagnostic and Therapeutic Difficulties. Eur J Case Rep Intern Med. 2018 Aug 28;5(8):000911. doi: 10.12890/2018_000911. PMID: 30756059; PMCID: PMC6346831.

12. WHO consolidated guidelines on treatment of Tuberculosis downloaded from https://www.who.int/publications/i/item/9789240048126 on 16072023.
13. Senderovitz T, Viskum K. Corticosteroids and tuberculosis. Resp med 1994;88:561–65.
14. Malik SK, Martin CS. Tuberculosis, corticosteroid therapy, and pulmonary function. Am Rev Respir Dis 1969;100:13–8.
15. Nemir RL, Cardona J, Vaziri F, Toledo R. Prednisone as an adjunct in the chemotherapy of lymph node—bronchial tuberculosis in childhood: a double blind study. Am Rev Respir Dis 1966; 402–410.
16. Vinod Kumar V. Unusual case of total lung collapse due to endobronchial TB—a case report. Apollo medicine (13):138–40.
17. Ryan H, Yoo J, Darsini P. Corticosteroids for tuberculous pleurisy. Cochrane Database Syst Rev [Internet]. 2017 [cited 2019 Sep 8];(3). Available from: https://www.cochranelibrary.com/cdsr/doi/10.1002/14651858.CD001876.pub3/ful.
18. Training module on extrapulmonary tuberculosis https://tbcindia.gov.in/showfile.php?lid=3679.
19. Kashyap S, Solanki A. Challenges in endobronchial tuberculosis: from diagnosis to management. Pulm Med 2014;2014:594806.
20. Toppet M, Malfroot A, Derde MP, et al. Corticosteroids in primary tuberculosis with bronchial obstruction. Arch Dis Child 1990;65:1222–6.
21. Rikimaru T. Therapeutic management of endobronchial tuberculosis. Expert Opin Pharmacother 2004;5:1463–70.
22. Neki NS. Endobronchial tuberculosis: an overview. Ann Pak Inst Med Sci 2013;9:105–9.
23. Kurasawa T, Kuze F, Kawai M, et al. Diagnosis and management of endobronchial tuberculosis. Intern Med 1992;31:593–8.
24. Training module on extrapulmonary tuberculosis. https://tbcindia.gov.in/showfile.php?lid=3681.
25. Gupta S, Ansari MAM, Gupta AK, Chaudhary P, Bansal LK. Current Approach for Diagnosis and Treatment of Adrenal Tuberculosis: Our Experience and Review of Literature. Surg J (N Y). 2022 Mar 3;8(1):e92–97. doi: 10.1055/s-0042-1743523. PMID: 35252566; PMCID: PMC8894089.
26. Bornstein SR, Allolio B, Arlt W. Diagnosis and treatment of primary adrenal insufficiency: an Endocrine Society Clinical Practice Guideline. J Clin Endocrinol Metab. 2016;101(02):364–89.
27. Huecker MR, Bhutta BS, Dominique E. Adrenal Insufficiency. [Updated 2023 Aug 17]. In: StatPearls [Internet]. Treasure Island (FL): StatPearls Publishing; 2024 Jan-. Available from: https://www.ncbi.nlm.nih.gov/books/NBK441832.
28. Nemir RL, Cardona J, Lacoius A, David M. Prednisone Therapy as an Adjunct in the Treatment of Lymph Node—Bronchial Tuberculosis in Childhood. A Double-Blind Study. Am Rev Respir Dis, 1963;88:189–98.
29. Gupta PR. Role of Add-on Prednisolone in the Management of Peripheral Lymph Node Tuberculosis. *J Infectiology*. 2018;1(2):4–6.
30. Schutz C, Davis AG, Sossen B, Lai RP, Ntsekhe M, Harley YX, Wilkinson RJ. Corticosteroids as an adjunct to tuberculosis therapy. Expert Rev Respir Med. 2018 Oct;12(10):881–891. doi: 10.1080/17476348.2018.1515628. Epub 2018 Sep 6. PMID: 30138039; PMCID: PMC6293474.
31. Bunkar ML, Agnihotri SP, Gupta PR, Arya S. Add-on prednisolone in the management of cervical lymph node tuberculosis. *Indian J Tuberc*, 2016;63(2):96–9.
32. Quinn CM, Poplin V, Kasibante J, Yuquimpo K, Gakuru J, Cresswell FV, Bahr NC. Tuberculosis IRIS: Pathogenesis, Presentation, and Management across the Spectrum of Disease. Life (Basel). 2020 Oct 29;10(11):262. doi: 10.3390/life10110262. PMID: 33138069; PMCID: PMC7693460.
33. Schutz C, Davis AG, Sossen B, Lai RP, Ntsekhe M, Harley YX, Wilkinson RJ. Corticosteroids as an adjunct to tuberculosis therapy. Expert Rev Respir Med. 2018 Oct;12(10):881–891. doi: 10.1080/17476348.2018.1515628. Epub 2018 Sep 6. PMID: 30138039; PMCID: PMC6293474.

Chapter

10

Steroids in Acute Respiratory Distress Syndrome and Sepsis

Samavedam Srinivas • Naveena Nayakanti

ACUTE RESPIRATORY DISTRESS SYNDROME (ARDS)

Acute respiratory distress syndrome (ARDS) is a life-threatening clinical syndrome characterized by arterial hypoxemia and heterogenous abnormalities anatomically and radiologically. The recognition of this condition has increased since the implementation of Berlin's definition.[1] This definition included the time frame of acute onset, PEEP requirement, and radiological features in defining the syndrome. Infections are the most common inciting events resulting in ARDS. The lung involvement in early ARDS is determined by inflammatory mediator-mediated alveolar damage, which damages the alveolar epithelium and impairs fluid resorption.[2] Phenotypes of ARDS with varying degrees of inflammatory activity have been recognised.[3]

Pathophysiology

The pathophysiology of ARDS is complex and is yet to be understood completely. The involvement of the inflammatory and coagulation pathways seems to be integral to the pathogenesis of ARDS. The evolution of the syndrome appears to occur over three overlapping stages—exudative, proliferative, and fibrotic.[4] All patients, however, do not pass through these stages mandatorily. The exudative phase is triggered by the initial insult and lasts for seven to ten days. This phase is characterized by the migration of the macrophages and neutrophils, which disrupt the endothelial and epithelial barriers during their migration. Inflammatory cells, fluid, protein, and red blood cells enter the airspace as a result of the disruption of the barriers. These events damage the type 1 and 2 alveolar pneumocytes with consequent loss of surfactant. In addition, the cellular debris gets deposited along the alveolar airspace. This accumulation of protein and cell-rich fluid produces a hyaline membrane, which is the histopathological hallmark of ARDS. This is followed by the proliferative phase, which lasts for a few weeks. This phase is reflective of the preparation for natural repair. This phase is mediated by anti-inflammatory cytokines and macrophages. Regeneration of pneumocytes and reestablishment of epithelial integrity are the events that occur during this phase. The last stage, the fibrotic stage, is seen only in a small percentage of patients, the reasons for which are still unclear. This is believed to be due to an excess of growth factors as the proliferative phase persists, resulting in the deposition of fibrotic tissue.

As is evident from the preceding discussion, inflammatory mechanisms and mediators play a major role in the pathogenesis of ARDS. As a result, steroids, with their known anti-inflammatory activity, have been extensively studied as therapeutic options for this condition. Corticosteroids are known anti-inflammatory agents and are implicated in numerous biological processes. The anti-inflammatory action is related to glucocorticoid activity and is mediated by both genomic and nongenomic signalling pathways. Their main mechanism of action is to inhibit the production of proinflammatory cytokines.[5]

The role of corticosteroids in the management of ARDS has been a subject of debate for a few decades.[6,7] The role of steroids in the management of ARDS can be compartmentalized into early use and late use. As discussed earlier, the initial stage of ARDS is characterized by alveolar inflammation. The potent anti-inflammatory action of glucocorticoids is expected to confer a theoretical benefit during this stage. Bernard et al in a multicenter randomised controlled trial (RCT), used a dose of 30 mg/kg of methyl prednisolone only for 24 hours among nearly 100 patients and failed to show a survival benefit.[8] Meduri et al, used a longer course of methylprednisolone, up to 32 days, in a very small cohort of patients and showed a benefit in terms of lung injury scores and survival.[9] Steinberg et al, working for the ARDS network, attempted to replicate the results from the Meduri trial, although for a shorter duration of therapy (14 days).[10] They used the same protocol as Meduri among 132 patients with early ARDS (7–13 days) and 180 patients with late ARDS (>13 days). The authors failed to show a survival benefit in either group. Annane, who has been a pioneer in studying steroid use in septic shock, evaluated the effect of hydrocortisone (50 mg IV 6 hourly) and Fludrocortisone (50 µg orally once a day) for a week in patients with ARDS.[11] The results were equivocal for the benefit of steroids on survival. Meduri attempted to replicate the results of his earlier study, on a larger sample size, at an earlier stage of ARDS (<72 hours) and succeeded in showing a statistically significant improvement in lung injury score and survival.[12] All these studies used the earlier AECC definition of ARDS.

The Berlin definition of ARDS came into vogue in 2012 and has been used as the eligibility criterion in studies published thereafter.[13] Villar et al were the first to evaluate the role of steroids in ARDS as per the Berlin definition.[14] They were also the first to study dexamethasone among patients with ARDS (moderate to severe). They used dexamethasone 20 mg once daily on days 1–5 and 10 mg once daily on days 6–10. They showed a significant difference in ventilator-free days on day 28 in the steroid group. They could not, however, show a survival benefit. The COVID pandemic in 2019 resulted in the evaluation of this particular class of steroids among patients with COVID-19 pneumonia. The RECOVERY trial, enrolling more than 6000 patients, used dexamethasone 6 mg daily for 10 days among all patients hospitalized for or with laboratory-confirmed COVID-19.[15] They showed a survival benefit with this regimen of corticosteroids, both among ventilated as well non-ventilated patients. Several other studies (REMAP-CAP[16] trial, CAPE COD,[17] and Met COVID[18] used hydrocortisone and methyl prednisolone for patients with varying severity of COVID-19 with varying results.

The use of corticosteroids in the late stages of ARDS was evaluated by the ARDS network group.[19] They evaluated the role of methylprednisolone in reducing 60-day mortality and ventilator-free days among 180 patients with ARDS of at least 7 days duration. The group could not show any benefit in survival or ventilator-free days when initiated more than 14 days after the onset of ARDS. The routine use of methylprednisolone cannot be recommended in the late stages of ARDS.

Conclusions

Based on current evidence, corticosteroids hold promise for improving outcomes in ARDS, particularly during the early stages. Viral pneumonia seems to respond positively to the use of steroids. Dexamethasone seems to be the most effective corticosteroid among those studied, demonstrating superior performance to methyl prednisolone or hydrocortisone. However, the timing of administration is crucial. Initiating corticosteroid therapy within the first week of ARDS onset appears to be most beneficial. Conversely, starting steroids after two weeks is linked to poorer patient outcomes. This emphasizes the importance of early intervention for maximizing the potential benefits of corticosteroids in ARDS management.

1. Corticosteroids have a theoretical benefit in the early stage of ARDS.
2. Viral pneumonia seems to respond positively to the use of steroids.
3. Dexamethasone seems to perform better than either methyl prednisolone or hydrocortisone.
4. Initiation should be considered within 7 days of the onset of ARDS.
5. Initiation of steroids after 14 days of onset of ARDS seems to be associated with adverse outcome.

STEROIDS IN SEPSIS

Sepsis is a life-threatening clinical condition with extensive physiological and biochemical abnormalities. The Third International Consensus (Sepsis 3) currently defines sepsis as "organ dysfunction caused by a dysregulated host response to infection", emphasizing for the first time the crucial role of the innate and adaptive immune response in the development of the clinical syndrome.[20] Septic shock, the most severe form, manifests with profound circulatory, metabolic, and cellular abnormalities. Management rests on prompt diagnosis, obtaining cultures, initiating broad-spectrum antibiotics, and addressing the source of infection. Supportive measures like vasoactive drugs and mechanical ventilation play a vital role. However, the utility of corticosteroids as an additional therapy for septic shock remains a topic of debate among intensivists. Despite several decades of research, inconsistent findings regarding mortality benefits across different trials have fuelled mixed opinions on their role.

Pathophysiology

Sepsis disrupts the delicate balance of pro- and anti-inflammatory pathways, triggering a cascade of cytokine and mediator release, activating coagulation and complement, and inducing tissue damage. Recognition of PAMPs and DAMPs by antigen-presenting cells and monocytes, facilitated by receptors like TLRs, initiates the cascade. This triggers NF-κB signalling, leading to "early activation gene" expression of proinflammatory mediators like IL-1, TNF-α, and interferons.[21] While anti-inflammatory pathways are concomitantly activated, the net response often leans towards hyperinflammation, characterized by increased cytokines, activated coagulation and complement, and tissue damage. This can ultimately culminate in multi-organ dysfunction. Later stages of sepsis witness immunosuppression via cell apoptosis and T cell exhaustion, rendering patients susceptible to opportunistic infections.[22]

Evidence

The first randomized trial exploring steroids in septic shock, conducted in 1976, showed promising results, which demonstrated improved mortality in septic shock patients receiving high-dose steroids (3 mg/kg dexamethasone or 30 mg/kg methylprednisolone). However, later studies employing high-dose steroids not only yielded inconsistent results regarding mortality benefits but also raised concerns about increased adverse events. This prompted a shift in research focus, leading to a deeper understanding of the complex interplay between corticosteroids and the pathophysiology of sepsis. In 2002, Annane et al conducted a ground-breaking study that divided septic shock patients into responders and non-responders to the corticotropin test. Their double-blinded, randomized trial compared low-dose hydrocortisone and fludrocortisone to placebo over seven days. Critically, the study found no significant mortality benefit for steroids in responders. However, in non-responders receiving low-dose therapy (50 mg hydrocortisone every 6 hours and 50 μg fludrocortisone daily), a significant reduction in 28-day mortality and vasopressor dependence was observed.[23] The CORTICUS trial by Sprung et al (2008) evaluated 50 mg intravenous hydrocortisone boluses every 6 hours with tapering on day 6 compared to placebo in septic shock patients. While hydrocortisone hastened shock reversal, it showed no improvement in 28-day survival.[24]

The 2016 Surviving Sepsis Campaign guidelines cautiously recommended the use of intravenous hydrocortisone if and only if fluid resuscitation and vasopressor therapy were unable to restore hemodynamic stability.[25] In a novel approach, the 2016 HYPRESS trial investigated whether early steroid intervention could prevent septic shock in patients with severe sepsis. This double-blinded, randomized controlled trial compared continuous hydrocortisone infusion (200 mg daily for 5 days, tapered to day 11) to placebo. While no significant differences were observed between groups in time to septic shock, ICU or hospital mortality, or 28-day mortality, the study was underpowered to definitively conclude. Notably, the hydrocortisone group exhibited increased hyperglycemia, but secondary infections, weaning failure, muscle weakness, hypernatremia, and other adverse events showed no significant difference.[26]

The clinical landscape for steroid use in septic shock shifted further in 2018 with publication of two large yet conflicting trials such as ADRENAL and APROCCHSS. ADRENAL, a double-blind RCT involving 3,800 patients with septic shock on mechanical ventilation, compared 7 days of continuous hydrocortisone infusion (200 mg daily) to placebo. Notably, while the trial found no difference in 90-day mortality between groups, hydrocortisone accelerated shock resolution and lowered blood transfusion requirements. However, 28-day mortality, shock recurrence, ICU/hospital length of stay, mechanical ventilation duration and recurrence, renal replacement therapy use, and new-onset bacteremia/fungemia remained statistically similar.[27] The multicenter, double-blind, randomized APROCCHSS trial assessed the impact of low-dose corticosteroids in septic shock. Patients received either hydrocortisone (50 mg IV bolus every 6 hours) combined with fludrocortisone (50 μg daily via nasogastric tube) or placebo. The study concluded that this 7-day regimen significantly reduced mortality at 90 days, as well as at ICU and hospital discharge, compared to placebo in adults with septic shock.[28]

The inconclusive evidence surrounding steroids in sepsis and septic shock has fuelled numerous meta-analyses. Notably, Liang et al, 2020 meta-analysis, encompassing 50 RCTs and over 12,000 patients, demonstrated no significant impact of corticosteroids on 28-day and long-term mortality, although a decrease in ICU and hospital mortality was observed.[29] Adding to the complexity, a recent retrospective study comparing hydrocortisone alone to hydrocortisone plus fludrocortisone in 653 septic shock patients found no difference in 90-day, 28-day, or in-hospital mortality between groups, along with no significant effect on length of hospital or ICU stay.[30]

With all this evidence and ongoing research, we still do not have guidelines with strong recommendations for steroids in sepsis and septic shock. While the use of corticosteroids (CS) in septic shock remains a subject of debate due to inconclusive evidence from various trials, most studies agree on their potential to shorten the duration of shock, ventilator dependence, and ICU stay. However, their administration should be strictly limited to adjunctive therapy for unresponsive cases only after adequate fluid resuscitation and vasopressor support.

Conclusion

While corticosteroids are not typically used for general sepsis, they can be a valuable tool in managing septic shock unresponsive to fluid resuscitation and requiring vasoactive medications. In such critical cases, hydrocortisone emerges as the preferred steroid, often administered as a 100 mg intravenous bolus followed by a maintenance dose of 50 mg every 6 hours or a continuous infusion at 10 mg/hr. This therapy continues until vasoactive agents can be gradually weaned off. Once hemodynamic stability is achieved, hydrocortisone is typically tapered over 2–3 days and then discontinued. It is crucial to remember that the benefits of corticosteroids are specific to septic shock with pneumonia or ARDS, and their use in other forms of sepsis requires separate evaluation. Additionally, close monitoring for potential side effects like hyperglycemia, high sodium levels (hypernatremia), increased risk of secondary infections, and other adverse events is essential throughout steroid therapy.

1. Steroids can be used in septic shock refractory to fluid resuscitation and requiring vasoactive agents.
2. Hydrocortisone is used as a 100 mg bolus followed by 50 mg every 6 hours or a continuous infusion at 10 mg/hr till vasoactive agents are weaned off.
3. Hydrocortisone is tapered over 2–3 days and stopped.
4. Steroids are not recommended in sepsis except for sepsis secondary to pneumonia and ARDS, which need to be discussed separately.
5. Monitor the patients for hyperglycemia, hypernatremia, secondary infections, and other adverse events while the patient is on steroids.

REFERENCES

1. Force ADT, Ranieri VM, Rubenfeld GD, Thompson B, Ferguson N, Caldwell E, Fan E, Camporota L, Slutsky AS. Acute respiratory distress syndrome: The Berlin Definition. JAMA 2012;307:2526–33.

2. Comparison of the Berlin Definition for Acute Respiratory Distress Syndrome with Autopsy—Pub Med. Available online:https://pubmed.ncbi.nlm.nih.gov/23370917/ (accessed on 7 January 2023).
3. Calfee CS, Delucchi K, Parsons PE, Thompson BT, Ware LB, Matthay MA. NHLBI ARDS Network. Sub-phenotypes in acute respiratory distress syndrome: Latent class analysis of data from two randomised controlled trials. Lancet Respir. Med. 2014;2:611–20.
4. Ramji HF, Hafiz M, Altaq HH, Hussain ST, Chaudry F. Acute Respiratory Distress Syndrome; A Review of Recent Updates and a Glance into the Future. Diagnostics (Basel). 2023 Apr 24;13(9):1528. doi: 10.3390/diagnostics13091528. PMID: 37174920; PMCID: PMC10177247.
5. Auphan N, DiDonato JA, Rosette C, Helmberg A, Karin M. Immunosuppression by glucocorticoids: Inhibition of NF-κB activity through induction of I kappa B synthesis. Science 1995;270:286–290.
6. Annane D. Pro: The illegitimate crusade against corticosteroids for severe H1N1 pneumonia. Am. *J. Respir. Crit. Care Med.* 2011;183:1125–26.
7. Matthay MA, Liu KD. Con: Corticosteroids are not indicated for the treatment of acute lung injury from H1N1 viral pneumonia. Am. J. Respir. Crit. Care Med. 2011;183:1127–28.
8. Bernard GR, Luce JM, Sprung CL, Rinaldo JE, Tate RM, Sibbald WJ, Kariman K, Higgins S, Bradley R, Metz CA. High-dose corticosteroids in patients with the adult respiratory distress syndrome. *N. Engl. J. Med.* 1987;317:1565–70.
9. Meduri GU, Headley AS, Golden E, Carson SJ, Umberger RA, Kelso T, Tolley EA. Effect of prolonged methylprednisolone therapy in un-resolving acute respiratory distress syndrome: A randomized controlled trial. JAMA 1998;280:159–65.
10. Steinberg KP, Hudson LD, Goodman RB, Hough CL, Lanken PN, Hyzy R, Thompson BT, Ancukiewicz M. National Heart, Lung, and Blood Institute Acute Respiratory Distress Syndrome (ARDS) Clinical Trials Network. Efficacy and safety of corticosteroids for persistent acute respiratory distress syndrome. *N. Engl. J. Med.* 2006;354:1671–84.
11. Annane D, Sébille V, Bellissant E, Ger-Inf-05 Study Group. Effect of low doses of corticosteroids in septic shock patients with or without early acute respiratory distress syndrome. Crit. Care Med. 2006;34:22–30.
12. Meduri GU, Golden E, Freire AX, Taylor E, Zaman M, Carson SJ, Gibson M, Umberger R. Methylprednisolone infusion in early severe ARDS: Results of a randomized controlled trial. Chest 2007;131:954–63.
13. Liufu R, Wang CY, Weng L, Du B. Newly Proposed Diagnostic Criteria for Acute Respiratory Distress Syndrome: Does Inclusion of High Flow Nasal Cannula Solve the Problem? J Clin Med. 2023 Jan 29;12(3):1043. doi: 10.3390/jcm12031043. PMID: 36769691; PMCID: PMC9917973.
14. Villar J, Ferrando C, Martínez D, Ambrós A, Muñoz T, Soler JA, Aguilar G, Alba F, González-Higueras E, Conesa LA. et al. Dexamethasone treatment for the acute respiratory distress syndrome: A multicentre, randomised controlled trial. Lancet Respir. Med. 2020;8:267–76.
15. RECOVERY Collaborative Group; Horby P, Lim WS, Emberson JR, Mafham M, Bell JL, Linsell L, Staplin N, Brightling C, Ustianowski A, et al. Dexamethasone in Hospitalized Patients with COVID-19. *N. Engl. J. Med.* 2021;384:693–704.
16. Angus DC, Derde L, Al-Beidh F, Annane D, Arabi Y, Beane A, van Bentum-Puijk W, Berry L, Bhimani Z, Bonten M, et al. Effect of Hydrocortisone on Mortality and Organ Support in Patients with Severe COVID-19: The REMAP-CAP COVID-19 Corticosteroid Domain Randomized Clinical Trial. JAMA 2020;324:1317–29.
17. Dequin PF, Meziani F, Quenot JP, Kamel T, Ricard J, Badie J, Reignier J, Heming N, Plantefève G, Souweine B, et al. Hydrocortisone in Severe Community-Acquired Pneumonia. N. Engl. J. Med. 2023.
18. Barros CMSS, Freire RS, Frota E, Rezende Santos AG, Farias MEL, Rodrigues MGA, Silva BM, Prado Jeronimo CM, Netto RLA, Silva Borba MG, et al. Short-Course of Methylprednisolone Improves Respiratory Functional Parameters After 120 Days in Hospitalized COVID-19 Patients (Metcovid Trial): A Randomized Clinical Trial. Front. Med. 2021;8:758405.

19. Steinberg KP, Hudson LD, Goodman RB, Hough CL, Lanken PN, Hyzy R, Thompson BT, Ancukiewicz M. Efficacy and safety of corticosteroids for persistent acute respiratory distress syndrome. *N Engl J Med* 2006;354:1671–84.
20. Singer M, Deutschman CS, Seymour CW, Shankar-Hari M, Annane D, Bauer M, et al. The third international consensus definitions for sepsis and septic shock (Sepsis 3). Jama. 2016;315:801–10. doi: 10.1001/jama.2016.0287.
21. Schulte W, Bernhagen J, and Bucala R, (2013). Cytokines in sepsis: potent immunoregulators and potential therapeutic targets—an updated view. Med. Inflamm. 2013:165974. doi: 10.1155/2013/165974.
22. Tamayo E, Fernandez A, Almansa R, Carrasco E, Heredia M, Lajo C, et al. Pro- and anti-inflammatory responses are regulated simultaneously from the first moments of septic shock. Europ Cytokine Netw. 2011;22:82–7. doi: 10.1684/ecn.2011.0281.
23. Annane D, Sébille V, Charpentier C, et al. Effect of Treatment with Low Doses of Hydrocortisone and Fludrocortisone on Mortality in Patients with Septic Shock. JAMA. 2002;288(7):862–71.
24. Sprung CL, Annane D, Keh D, Moreno R, Singer M, Freivogel K, et al. Hydrocortisone therapy for patients with septic shock. N Engl J Med. 2008;358:111–24. doi: 10.1056/NEJMoa071366.
25. RhodesA, EvansLE, AlhazzaniW, et al. Surviving Sepsis Campaign: international guidelines for the management of sepsis and septic shock. Intensive Care Med. 2017;43(3):304–77. doi:10.1007/s00134-017-4683-6.
26. Keh D, Trips E, Marx G, et al. Effect of Hydrocortisone on Development of Shock Among Patients With Severe Sepsis: The HYPRESS Randomized Clinical Trial. JAMA. 2016;316(17):1775–85.
27. Venkatesh B, Finfer S, Cohen J, et al. Adjunctive Glucocorticoid Therapy in Patients with Septic Shock. *N Engl J Med.* 2018;378(9):797–808.
28. Annane D, Renault A, Brun-Buisson C, et al. Hydrocortisone Plus Fludrocortisone for Adults with Septic Shock. *N Engl J Med.* 2018;378:809–18.
29. Liang H, Song H, Zhai R, Song G, Li H, Ding X, Kan Q, and Sun T. Corticosteroids for Treating Sepsis in Adult Patients: A Systematic Review and Meta-Analysis. Front. Immunol. 2021;12:709155. doi: 10.3389/fimmu.2021.709155.
30. Cheng X, Fu Z, Liu Y, Zheng X, and Hu T. Association of mortality with fludrocortisone addition to hydrocortisone treatment among septic shock patients: a propensity score matching analysis. Front. Med. 2023;10:1190758. doi: 10.3389/fmed.2023.1190758.

Chapter 11

Steroids in Eosinophilic Lung Diseases

M Ramakrishna Reddy • G Uma Sri

INTRODUCTION

Pulmonary eosinophilia (PE) signifies an abnormal accumulation of eosinophils within the lung compartments, constituting the airways, interstitium, and alveoli. Diverse etiologies, including infections, parasites, medications, autoimmune conditions, malignancies, and obstructive lung diseases, can trigger this influx of eosinophils. Consequently, PE is broadly categorized into two main groups: Primary (idiopathic) PE and secondary PE. The causative agent remains elusive in primary PE, manifesting as entities like acute eosinophilic pneumonia (AEP), chronic eosinophilic pneumonia (CEP), hypereosinophilic syndrome (HES), and eosinophilic granulomatosis with polyangiitis (EGPA). Secondary PE arises from identifiable causes such as parasitic infections, allergic bronchopulmonary aspergillosis (ABPA), drug reactions, radiation exposure, and malignancies. Recognizing this dichotomy in etiology is crucial for guiding accurate diagnosis and effective management of PE.

EOSINOPHILIC PNEUMONIA

Eosinophilic pneumonia (EP) is a clinical term defined by the presence of pulmonary infiltrates on imaging, peripheral blood eosinophilia, and alveolar eosinophil presence confirmed by bronchoalveolar lavage (BAL) or lung biopsy. This spectrum further divides into acute eosinophilic pneumonia (AEP), characterized by rapid onset and potential respiratory failure, and chronic eosinophilic pneumonia (CEP), with a more insidious course and variable respiratory symptoms.

Acute Eosinophilic Pneumonia

Acute eosinophilic pneumonia (AEP), an idiopathic eosinophilic lung disease, presents abruptly with features mimicking ARDS, posing a significant diagnostic dilemma due to absent peripheral eosinophilia. A history of recent smoking changes (initiation, brand switch, e-cigarettes) or heavy dust/sand exposure should raise suspicion.[1] Bronchoalveolar lavage demonstrating >25% eosinophils confirms the diagnosis. High-resolution CT findings (ground-glass opacities, septal thickening, pleural effusions) may overlap with ARDS, but lung biopsy reveals the definitive picture with marked eosinophilic infiltration alongside diffuse alveolar damage and interstitial edema. This constellation of features, despite the atypical lack of peripheral eosinophilia, points towards AEP diagnosis.

Management of AEP

Management of AEP primarily hinges on identifying and addressing the underlying cause. For cases linked to exogenous exposures like tobacco smoke or medications, the cornerstone of therapy involves eliminating the offending agent and initiating systemic glucocorticoids.[2] Idiopathic AEP is also similarly treated with systemic glucocorticoids. While some patients with milder disease may improve solely with exposure cessation and no steroids, more severe cases may require supportive measures like supplemental oxygen and even mechanical ventilation in a hospital setting. AEP related to infections requires the identification of the culprit microorganism and administer appropriate antimicrobial therapy.[3]

The optimal corticosteroid regimen for AEP remains elusive, lacking a standardized protocol. Clinical practice often dictates the initial dose based on disease severity. In hospitalized patients with critical hypoxemic respiratory failure necessitating mechanical ventilation, intravenous methylprednisolone (60–125 mg every 6 hours) is commonly used. Upon respiratory improvement and successful extubation (typically within 1–3 days), the therapy may transition to oral prednisone for up to 6–12 weeks.[4] In presentations without initial respiratory failure, oral prednisone at 40–60 mg daily is usually initiated and progressively tapered over 2–6 weeks, guided by the rate of symptom and objective improvement, including oxygen saturation and radiographic findings.[5] Interestingly, recent studies by RHEE et al suggest that 2 weeks of corticosteroid therapy for patients with respiratory failure may be just as effective as 4 weeks.[6] This shorter duration offers promising potential for equal efficacy, with a majority achieving major symptom resolution within 3 days. The overall prognosis of AEP is excellent upon treatment, with resolution of radiologic infiltrates and no long-term pulmonary sequelae (For specific steroid dosing recommendations on AEP please refer to Table 11.1).

Chronic Eosinophilic Pneumonia

Chronic eosinophilic pneumonia (CEP) is an idiopathic interstitial lung disease (ILD) characterized by persistent eosinophilic inflammation and infiltration of the lung's

Table 11.1: Glucocorticoid dosing in acute eosinophilic pneumonia (AEP)

Severity	*Initial dose*	*Route*	*Duration*	*Tapering*
Mild	None	N/A	N/A	N/A
Moderate (no initial respiratory failure)	Prednisone 40–60 mg daily	Oral	2–6 weeks	Gradual, based on symptom and objective improvement
Severe (hypoxemic respiratory failure and MV support)	Methylprednisolone 60–125 mg every 6 hours	IV	1–3 days	Transition to oral prednisone 40–60 mg daily for 6–12 weeks upon extubation

interstitial and alveolar spaces. This often presents with peripheral blood eosinophilia and a history of underlying asthma. Patients typically experience a gradual progression of cough, fever, shortness of breath (dyspnea), and wheezing over weeks to months. Chest imaging reveals a characteristic pattern, termed the "photographic negative of pulmonary edema," exhibiting bilateral peripheral pleural-based opacities.[7] A definitive diagnosis hinges on bronchoalveolar lavage (BAL), revealing a predominance of eosinophils exceeding 40% of the leukocyte count. Additionally, both BAL and lung biopsy are useful in excluding alternative causes, such as drug-induced or infectious etiologies.

Management of CEP

CEP exhibits a remarkable response to corticosteroids, with rapid clinical improvement often seen within 48 hours. Despite an excellent overall prognosis, relapses occur frequently during corticosteroid tapering, highlighting the need for individualized therapy based on disease severity. While no standardized guidelines exist, typical initial therapy involves oral prednisone at 1 mg/kg/day for 4–6 weeks, followed by gradual tapering[8] (Table 11.2). However, a significant challenge arises with relapse rates reaching up to 80% upon cessation of steroids. To address this issue, maintenance therapy with slowly tapered prednisone over 6–12 months is often employed. Additionally, targeted agents like omalizumab (anti-IgE), mepolizumab (anti-IL-5), benralizumab, and reslizumab (anti-IL-5) have shown success in case reports, offering promising avenues for future management.[9–12]

Table 11.2: Corticosteroid treatment regimens for CEP

Treatment phase	*Dose*	*Duration*	*Tapering*
Initial therapy	Prednisone 1 mg/kg/day	4–6 weeks	Gradual
Maintenance therapy	Prednisone (dose adjusted based on response)	6–12 months	Gradual

DRUG-INDUCED EOSINOPHILIC PNEUMONIA

DIEP's clinical heterogeneity manifests in two principal forms: Acute and subacute/chronic. The acute form, accounting for around 70% of cases, presents remarkably similar to idiopathic AEP. In contrast, the subacute/chronic form, affecting roughly 30% of patients, clinically overlaps with idiopathic CEP. A hallmark feature of DIEP is marked peripheral eosinophilia, >1000 cells/ml, serving as a strong suggestive indicator of drug-induced etiology.

A literature review of case reports identified daptomycin, minocycline, and nitrofurantoin among antibiotics, and mesalamine and sulfasalazine among anti-inflammatory agents, emerged as the top five offenders, collectively accounting for more than 50% of DIEP cases.[13]

While specific tests like drug-specific lymphocyte transformation assays can support the identification of an offending agent, the pillar of management in DIEP lies in pinpointing and discontinuing the culprit drug. Corticosteroids are the primary treatment for drug-induced eosinophilia, aiming to resolve both clinical symptoms and radiologic infiltrates. Fortunately, the dose and duration of this therapy are similar to those used for idiopathic acute eosinophilic pneumonia (AEP). Notably, unlike chronic eosinophilic pneumonia, DIEP typically requires only months of corticosteroid therapy.

Furthermore, the risk of relapse following steroid tapering is rare in drug-induced cases, offering a distinct prognosis compared to its idiopathic counterpart.

STEROIDS IN HYPEREOSINOPHILIC SYNDROMES

HES encompasses a heterogeneous group of disorders defined by persistent peripheral blood eosinophilia exceeding $1.5 \times 10^9/L$, independent of secondary causes, and manifesting with eosinophil-mediated organ damage.[14] Three main subtypes exist such as myeloid variant (M-HES), lymphocytic variant (L-HES), and the rare familial variant (HESFA).

M-HES arises from a chromosome 4q deletion, leading to the formation and expression of the FIP1L1-PDGFRA fusion gene.[15] Other, less frequent chromosomal rearrangements involving PDGFRA or PDGFRB and alternative fusion partners like FGFR1 and JAK2 can also contribute to M-HES. In contrast, L-HES originates from clonal expansion of CD4 T cells lacking surface T cell receptor (TCR)/CD3 complex expression, leading to elevated type 2 cytokine production and subsequent hypereosinophilia. The most recognized example of L-HES is the CD3–CD4+ T cell-associated subtype.

The skin, lungs, and gastrointestinal tract are the primary targets of HES. Respiratory involvement is a prominent feature of HES, with frequent complaints of cough, dyspnea, and wheezing. These symptoms, along with pulmonary infiltrates on imaging, often mimic asthma or acute respiratory failure. However, the presence of eosinophilia and lack of response to conventional asthma therapy warrants further investigation for HES.

Management of HES

For patients with the FIP1L1-PDGFRA fusion gene, prompt initiation of imatinib mesylate is crucial, as this targeted tyrosine kinase inhibitor directly inhibits the abnormal protein product.[15] Additionally, administration of oral prednisolone at 1 mg/kg/day for a few days is recommended to mitigate potential sequelae of mass eosinophil degranulation during initial treatment.

For all other patients with HES (patients lacking the FIP1L1-PDGFRA fusion or other imatinib-responsive mutations, lymphoid HES, and idiopathic HES), corticosteroids represent first-line therapy with a very high response rate. A regimen of prednisolone, 1 mg/kg/day for several weeks, is typically followed by gradual tapering to an every-other-day schedule once disease stabilization is achieved. Long-term continuation for approximately one year is generally recommended (Table 11.3).

Patients with HES exhibiting corticosteroid resistance or unacceptable long-term dependence require consideration of alternative therapeutic options. Hydroxyurea, interferon-α (standard or pegylated), cyclosporine A, alemtuzumab, and various cytotoxic agents represent potential second-line options, each with unique benefits and limitations. While their efficacy varies, often falling within the 20–60% success rate range, and is often limited by poor tolerability and safety concerns (e.g. cytopenias with hydroxyurea, infections with interferon-α), these agents still offer valuable tools for managing difficult-to-treat HES. Due to the diversity of efficacy, tolerability, and safety profiles, careful patient assessment and close monitoring are paramount for optimal selection and administration of second-line therapy in HES, ensuring safe and effective outcomes.

Table 11.3: Management of hypereosinophilic syndromes (HES)

HES variant	*Initial therapy*	*Maintenance therapy*	*Duration*
FIP1L1-PDGFRA fusion positive	Imatinib mesylate 100 mg per day + Prednisolone 1 mg/kg/day (first few days only)	Imatinib mesylate maintenance dose	Until sustained remission
FIP1L1-PDGFRA fusion negative (no imatinib response), lymphoid HES and idiopathic HES	Prednisolone 1 mg/kg/day	Prednisolone tapered to every-other-day schedule	Approximately 1 year
Corticosteroid-resistant or severe cases	Individualized based on response and tolerability	Hydroxyurea, interferon-α, cyclosporine A, and alemtuzumab	As needed

EOSINOPHILIC GRANULOMATOSIS WITH POLYANGIITIS (EGPA)

EGPA, formerly known as allergic angiitis with granulomatosis or Churg-Strauss syndrome, is a rare and potentially fatal systemic vasculitis characterized by a characteristic clinical triad: Chronic asthma, tissue eosinophilia, and small vessel vasculitis. Approximately 40% of EGPA patients exhibit antineutrophil cytoplasmic antibodies (ANCA), placing them within the spectrum of pulmonary ANCA-associated vasculitides.

Treatment

In eosinophilic granulomatosis with polyangiitis (EGPA), treatment is guided by the severity of the disease. The French Vasculitis Study Group's Five Factor Score (FFS) serves as a valuable prognostic tool, guiding therapeutic decisions. Corticosteroids, specifically oral prednisone starting at 1 mg/kg/day for 3–4 weeks followed by a gradual taper to 5–10 mg/day by 1 year, serve as the cornerstone of EGPA treatment. In critically ill patients, an initial methylprednisolone bolus (15 mg/kg/day for 1–3 days) may be necessary.[16] However, for those unresponsive to or relapsing on corticosteroids, steroid-sparing strategies come into play.

For severe presentations with potential for life-threatening complications, cyclophosphamide (0.6–0.7 g/m^2 intravenously at days 1, 15, and 30, then every 3 weeks) is added to corticosteroids to induce remission.[17] In refractory cases, various options like subcutaneous interferon-α, high-dose intravenous immunoglobulins, plasma exchange, cyclosporine, and rituximab have shown success, highlighting the need for individualized treatment approaches based on patient response and disease severity.

For an in-depth exploration of EGPA treatment, please refer to the CTD ILD chapter in this book, addressing crucial topics like achieving remission, maintaining it, managing relapses and resistant cases, and handling EGPA in specific circumstances.

ALLERGIC BRONCHOPULMONARY ASPERGILLOSIS (ABPA/ABPM)

Allergic bronchopulmonary aspergillosis (ABPA) is a complex airway disease characterized by type I and III hypersensitivity reactions to *Aspergillus* species. Diagnosis relies on multiple criteria, with the recent International Society for Human and Animal Mycology (ISHAM) criteria setting a higher total serum IgE cut-off (1000 IU/ml) for improved specificity. A comprehensive evaluation for ABPA typically involves measuring total serum IgE, Aspergillus-specific IgE, and IgG antibodies, performing Aspergillus skin prick tests, detecting Aspergillus precipitins in serum via immunoelectrophoresis and CT chest to assess for potential bronchiectasis.

Corticosteroids constitute the mainstay of therapy for ABPA, targeting both eosinophilic inflammation and allergic components. While systemic administration is well-established, optimal dosing and duration remain debated. One common approach (Greenberger, 2002) involves initial prednisolone 0.5 mg/kg/day for 2 weeks, followed by 0.5 mg/kg every other day for 6–8 weeks, then further tapering by 5–10 mg every 2 weeks with discontinuation at 3 months.[18] Alternative regimens, such as Agarwal et al high-dose protocol of prednisolone 0.75 mg/kg/day for 6 weeks, then 0.5 mg/kg/day for 6 weeks, followed by a tapering dose to 5 mg every 6 weeks to continue for a total duration of 6–12 months are also employed.[19] Recent randomized controlled trials demonstrate no significant clinical difference between medium (initial 0.5 mg/kg/day prednisolone for 2 weeks) and high-dose (initial 0.75 mg/kg/day prednisolone for 6 weeks) corticosteroid regimens.

Oral itraconazole 200 mg twice daily for 4–6 months, tapered over the next 4–6 months, serves as a valuable adjunct to corticosteroids. This antifungal therapy reduces fungal burden in the lungs, enabling corticosteroid dose reduction and minimizing exacerbation frequency.[20] In ABPA patients with severe or refractory asthma, the anti-IgE recombinant antibody omalizumab may also be considered.

EOSINOPHILIC PNEUMONIA IN PARASITIC DISEASES

Parasitic infections remain the primary driver of eosinophilic pneumonia (EP) globally. Among these, simple pulmonary eosinophilia, also known as Loeffler syndrome, manifests as a mild form of EP characterized by transient cough, wheezing, fever, elevated blood eosinophil counts, and fleeting pulmonary infiltrates. Transmission in Ascaris-induced EP occurs *via* the faecal–oral route, while Strongyloides employs a distinct strategy, directly penetrating the skin to reach the intestine. Both parasites mature in the gut, releasing eggs that hatch into larvae. These larvae then migrate through the venous circulation to the lungs, triggering pulmonary symptoms through their movement within the bronchial and tracheal tree before ultimately being swallowed and completing their cycle in the small intestine. Ascariasis readily succumbs to oral mebendazole or albendazole, while ivermectin effectively combats Strongyloides infection.[21] In tropical regions, filarial parasites *Wuchereria bancrofti* and *Brugia malayi* cause tropical pulmonary eosinophilia, with diethylcarbamazine serving as the mainstay of treatment.

Visceral larva migrans (VLM) syndrome, primarily triggered by the larval migration of *Toxocara canis* (dog roundworm) or *Toxocara cati* (cat roundworm), manifests with a constellation of symptoms including fever, seizures, fatigue, pronounced blood eosinophilia, and transient pulmonary findings like cough, dyspnea, wheezing, crackles on auscultation, and fleeting pulmonary infiltrates on chest X-ray. While VLM often demonstrates a self-limiting course, moderate to severe cases benefit from effective therapy with albendazole for 5 days alongside judicious corticosteroid administration.

RADIATION PNEUMONITIS

Concurrent chemoradiotherapy, a frequently employed modality in thoracic malignancies, carries an increased risk of radiotherapy-induced lung injury (RILI) compared to monotherapy. RILI manifests in two distinct phases: Radiation pneumonitis occurs within weeks to months after treatment, while radiation fibrosis develops over months to years. Radiation pneumonitis is characterized by direct cytotoxic effects of ionizing radiation, oxidative stress-induced secondary damage, immune-mediated injury, and subsequent radiation fibrosis.

Accurate RP diagnosis hinges on comprehensive clinical correlation and thorough exclusion of frequent mimics like disease progression and infection. Despite the absence of substantial data, systemic corticosteroids, typically prednisolone at 0.5–1 mg/kg/day for 2 weeks followed by a gradual taper, currently serve as the cornerstone of therapy for acute pneumonitis.[22] Their efficacy lies in reducing inflammation and curtailing TNF-mediated endothelial and lymphocyte injury.

Conclusion

Glucocorticosteroids are a mainstay in the treatment of various eosinophilic lung diseases due to their potent anti-inflammatory properties. In idiopathic entities like AEP and CEP, corticosteroids effectively control symptoms and induce remission, although relapses are frequent in CEP, necessitating steroid-sparing agents. Conversely, drug-induced eosinophilic pneumonia (DIEP) typically necessitates shorter corticosteroid courses with a lower relapse risk. In HES, corticosteroids represent first-line therapy for most variants, with imatinib specifically targeting the FIP1L1-PDGFRA fusion gene mutation. In EGPA, corticosteroids are often combined with cyclophosphamide for disease induction and maintenance, whereas ABPA management involves corticosteroids alongside antifungal medications like itraconazole. While the optimal corticosteroid regimen varies across diseases, their role in mitigating eosinophilic inflammation and associated clinical manifestations remains central to the therapeutic approach in eosinophilic lung diseases.

REFERENCES

1. De Giacomi F, Vassallo R, Yi ES, et al. Acute eosinophilic pneumonia. causes, diagnosis, and management. *Am J Respir Crit Care Med* 2018;197:728–36.
2. Salahuddin, M., Anjum, F. and Cherian, S.V., 2017. Pulmonary Eosinophilia.
3. Allen J, Wert M. Eosinophilic Pneumonias. *The Journal of Allergy and Clinical Immunology*. In practice. 2018 Sep–Oct:6(5):1455–61.
4. Allen JN, Pacht ER, Gadek JE, et al. Acute eosinophilic pneumonia is a reversible cause of noninfectious respiratory failure. *N Engl J Med* 1989;321:569–74.
5. Allen J. Acute eosinophilic pneumonia. Seminars in Respiratory and Critical Care Medicine. 2006;27(2).

6. Rhee CK, Min KH, Yim NY, et al. Clinical characteristics and corticosteroid treatment of acute eosinophilic pneumonia. *Eur Respir J* 2013;41:402–9.
7. Janahi IA, Rehman A, Baloch NUA. Corticosteroids and their use in Respiratory Disorders [Internet]. Corticosteroids. In Tech; 2018. Available from: http://dx.doi.org/10.5772/intechopen.72147.
8. Marchand E, Reynaud-Gaubert M, Lauque D, Durieu J, Tonnel AB, Cordier JF. Idiopathic chronic eosinophilic pneumonia. A clinical and follow-up study of 62 cases. The Groupe d'Etudes et de Recherche sur les Maladies "Orphelines" Pulmonaires (GERM"O"P) Medicine (Baltimore) 1998;77:299–312.
9. Kaya H, Gumus S, Ucar E, et al. Omalizumab as a steroid-sparing agent in chronic eosinophilic pneumonia. Chest 2012;142:513–6.
10. Brenard E, Pilette C, Dahlqvist C, et al. Real-life study of mepolizumab in idiopathic chronic eosinophilic pneumonia. Lung 2020;198:355–60.
11. Sarkis E, Patel S, Burns K, et al. Anti-interleukin (IL)-5 as a steroid-sparing agent in chronic eosinophilic pneumonia. *J Asthma* 2020;57:82–6.
12. Fowler C, Hoover W. Dupilumab for chronic eosinophilic pneumonia. Pediatr Pulmonol 2020;55: 3229–30.
13. Bartal C, Sagy I, Barski L. Drug-induced eosinophilic pneumonia: a review of 196 case reports. Medicine (Baltimore) 2018;97:e9688.
14. Chusid MJ, Dale DC, West BC, Wolff SM. The hypereosinophilic syndrome: analysis of fourteen cases with review of the literature. Medicine (Baltimore) 1975;54:1–27.
15. Cools J, DeAngelo DJ, Gotlib J, et al. A tyrosine kinase created by a fusion of the PDGFRA and FIP1L1 genes as a therapeutic target of imatinib in idiopathic hypereosinophilic syndrome. *N Engl J Med* 2003;348:1201–14.
16. Dunogue´ B, Pagnoux C, Guillevin L. Churg-Strauss syndrome: clinical symptoms, complementary investigations, prognosis and outcome, and treatment. Semin Respir Crit Care Med 2011;32:298–309.
17. Guillevin L, Pagnoux C, Seror R, et al. The Five Factor Score revisited: assessment of prognoses of systemic necrotizing vasculitides based on the French Vasculitis Study Group (FVSG) cohort. Medicine (Baltimore) 2011;90:19–27.
18. Greenberger PA. Allergic bronchopulmonary aspergillosis. J Allergy Clin Immunol. 2002;110: 685–92.
19. Agarwal R. Allergic bronchopulmonary aspergillosis. Chest. 2009;135:805–26.
20. Agarwal R. What is the current place of azoles in allergic bronchopulmonary aspergillosis and severe asthma with fungal sensitization? Expert Rev Respir Med. 2012;6:363–71.
21. Salahuddin M, Anjum F, Cherian SV. Pulmonary Eosinophilia. [Updated 2023 May 22]. In: StatPearls [Internet]. Treasure Island (FL): StatPearls Publishing; 2024 Jan-. Available from: https://www.ncbi.nlm.nih.gov/books/NBK470600/
22. Jain V, Berman AT. Radiation pneumonitis: old problem, new tricks. Cancers (Basel). 2018;10(7):1.

Chapter

12

Steroids in Lung Malignancy

Deepak Koppaka • Pragna Sagar Rapole • Naren Bolineni, Satish

INTRODUCTION

Lung cancer stands as the most prevalent cancer worldwide, responsible for a significant number of cancer-related deaths globally.[1] Traditional treatment modalities like surgery, radiotherapy, and chemotherapy have long been the mainstays in the management of this disease. Over the last decade, the introduction of novel therapies, including targeted therapies and immunotherapies, has revolutionized lung cancer management and improved patient outcomes significantly. Amid these advancements, the role of steroids in the treatment of lung cancer has come under scrutiny, particularly with the emergence of immunotherapy as a promising therapeutic approach. This chapter explores the role of steroids in the prevention and management of lung cancer, considering their historical significance and potential implications in the context of modern treatment strategies (Fig. 12.1).

CHEMOPREVENTION

Patients with chronic obstructive pulmonary disease (COPD) have a markedly elevated risk of developing lung cancer due to the persistent chronic inflammation in this

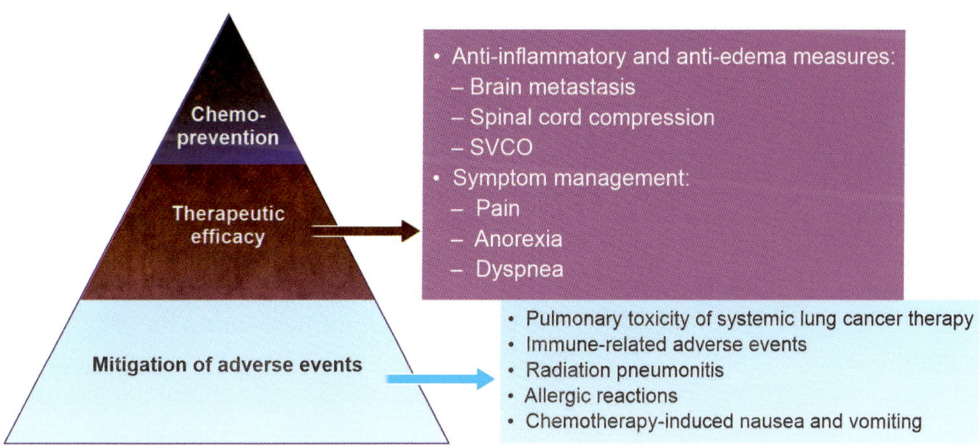

Fig. 12.1: Role of steroids in the prevention and management of lung cancer

condition.[2] As a potential countermeasure, inhalational corticosteroids (ICS) have been proposed as agents that could mitigate inflammation, consequently reducing the associated cancer risk.[3]

However, the role of inhalational steroids in COPD patients as a means of chemoprevention remains a topic of ongoing debate. While there is a plausible rationale for their use in lowering inflammation-associated cancer risks, the effectiveness of inhalational steroids in achieving this goal remains uncertain.

Furthermore, the question of a potential dose–response relationship between ICS exposure and cancer risk reduction is unanswered. Determining the optimal dosage, frequency, and duration of inhalational steroid use necessary to achieve a meaningful reduction in lung cancer risk in COPD patients remains a point of active investigation and contention.

THERAPEUTIC EFFICACY

Steroids play a vital role in the management of lymphomas and leukemias. They possess a preferential lymphocytolytic activity, by inducing apoptosis, or programmed cell death, in lymphoid cell populations. These properties make steroids indispensable in the treatment of non-Hodgkins lymphomas, acute and chronic lymphoblastic lymphoma/leukemia, and myelomas. Moreover, steroids offer therapeutic benefits that extend beyond their cytolytic effects. In lung cancer management, steroids are employed for their anti-inflammatory, and anti-edema properties, and to control symptoms.

Anti-inflammatory and Anti-edema Properties

Brain Metastasis

Lung cancers account for nearly 40–65% of secondary brain tumours.[4] Patients with brain metastasis frequently experience a decline in quality of life and neurological functions. Steroids offer relief by improving quality of life and alleviating neurological symptoms. In cases where brain metastasis causes symptoms due to mass effect, corticosteroids, with dexamethasone being the preferred choice, are recommended.[5] Dosing depends on symptom severity, ranging from 4–8 mg/day for mild symptoms to higher doses of up to 16 mg/day for moderate to severe symptoms. Dose tapering should align with clinical tolerance and where possible should be rapid. Steroids have a limited role in asymptomatic brain metastasis without mass effect.

The QUARTZ study, a non-inferiority trial in non-small cell lung cancer (NSCLC), examined whether brain radiotherapy in addition to steroids and supportive care improves quality of life and overall survival.[6] The dose of dexamethasone was adjusted based on symptom response. Interestingly, the study found that the addition of whole-brain radiotherapy (WBRT) to steroids and best supportive care did not yield additional benefits. This suggests that in patients with multiple brain metastases, poor performance status, elderly NSCLC, and limited life expectancy, steroids coupled with best supportive care may be as effective as adding WBRT, without notable additional improvements in relevant parameters.

Spinal Cord Compression

Spinal cord compression is a critical medical condition where steroids play a pivotal role in treatment. Steroids are instrumental in reducing vasogenic edema and inflammation, while also stabilizing vascular membranes. By addressing these factors, steroids contribute to decreasing subsequent occurrences of ischemia, infarction, and irreversible damage at the compressed spinal cord site.[7]

A significant advantage of steroid administration is the rapid improvement it can induce in motor function, especially when initiated within the first 12 hours of symptoms. This improvement serves as a positive prognostic indicator, as it is correlated with further strength recovery after definitive treatment. Typically, this immediate treatment with steroids is followed by the initiation of definitive treatments, such as radiotherapy or surgical stabilization.

The dosing and duration of steroid administration vary among studies. Based on available evidence, an initial intravenous bolus of 10 mg dexamethasone, followed by 16 mg orally once daily, has demonstrated fewer complications compared to higher initial bolus doses and prolonged oral dosing.[7] After definitive treatment, a rapid weaning process for steroids is recommended.

Superior Vena Cava Obstruction (SVCO)

The anti-inflammatory properties of steroids are essential in situations such as airway compression and SVCO.[8] While there are no randomised studies evaluating the benefit of steroids in patients with SVCO, most guidelines continue to recommend steroids in patients with SVCO. When steroids are used they are recommended in high doses and for a shorter duration.

Symptom Management

Pain

Pain is a prevalent and distressing symptom among patients with lung cancer. Addressing pain in these patients typically follows the World Health Organization (WHO) analgesic ladder, with opioids being a cornerstone of pain management. Corticosteroids demonstrate efficacy in relieving pain associated with space-occupying lesions, where factors like inflammation and edema contribute to discomfort within confined areas.[9]

Corticosteroids have emerged as potential complements to pain management due to their effects on all stages of pain nociception: Transduction, transmission, modulation, and pain perception. With their anti-inflammatory properties and the ability to reduce vascular permeability, steroids function as adjunctive treatments for pain reduction.

The quality of the evidence for the efficacy of corticosteroids for pain control in cancer patients is weak.[10] Although some studies report noteworthy pain relief with corticosteroids, these effects tend to be transient. Dexamethasone is the most frequently employed corticosteroid in pain management. It offers the advantage of reduced fluid retention compared to other steroids, attributable to its diminished mineralocorticoid impact.

Anorexia

Cancer-related anorexia leading to cachexia is prevalent in advanced lung cancer patients. This condition not only compromises treatment tolerance but also linked to decreased survival rates. Presently, there are only two approved treatments for anorexia: Progestins and corticosteroids.[11,12]

In patients with advanced cancer administering 4 mg of dexamethasone twice daily for 14 days has exhibited positive outcomes, with notable improvements in fatigue and anorexia. However, these improvements tend to be short-lived, with studies indicating no positive effects on lean body mass.[13] Furthermore, the prolonged use of corticosteroids can exacerbate proximal myopathy, a condition characterized by muscle weakness in the upper arms and thighs.

Given these considerations, the use of dexamethasone for appetite stimulation seems most appropriate for short-term utilization, particularly in patients nearing the end of life. While it can provide temporary relief from symptoms like fatigue and anorexia its extended application may not yield significant benefits.

Dyspnea

Dyspnea, commonly referred to as air hunger, encompasses a range of breathing discomfort sensations that vary in intensity. This subjective experience is a prevalent and distressing symptom, particularly affecting patients with advanced lung cancer. Its prevalence and intensity tend to increase as patients near the final weeks or days of life.

To manage dyspnea, both non-pharmacological and pharmacological approaches are available. Steroids find utility in cases where airway obstruction or inflammation significantly contributes to dyspnea. In these scenarios, short-term systemic corticosteroid administration is common. Dexamethasone, usually dosed at 8–16 mg per day for 1–2 weeks, is frequently employed for this purpose.[14]

Notably, dexamethasone has shown efficacy not only in addressing dyspnea but also in alleviating radiation-induced pain flare. While the evidence is relatively limited, several small case reports or series have suggested that corticosteroids may hold particular promise in managing conditions like central airway obstruction, lymphangitic carcinomatosis, and superior vena cava syndrome, where these conditions contribute to the dyspnea experienced by patients.[15]

MITIGATING ADVERSE EVENTS

Pulmonary Toxicity of Systemic Lung Cancer Therapy

The administration of systemic therapies in the management of lung cancer brings with it a spectrum of potential pulmonary toxicities. This pertains to all three categories of agents used: Chemotherapy, targeted therapy, and immunotherapy. Hypersensitivity reaction, apoptotic dysfunction or impaired repair processes are the most common mechanisms underlying drug-induced lung damage. Pneumonitis can be classified into several categories based on clinicoradiographic and histopathologic features, including nonspecific interstitial pneumonitis, organizing pneumonia, hypersensitivity pneumonitis, diffuse alveolar damage/acute respiratory distress syndrome, diffuse alveolar hemorrhage, and eosinophilic pneumonia. Chemotherapy-induced lung

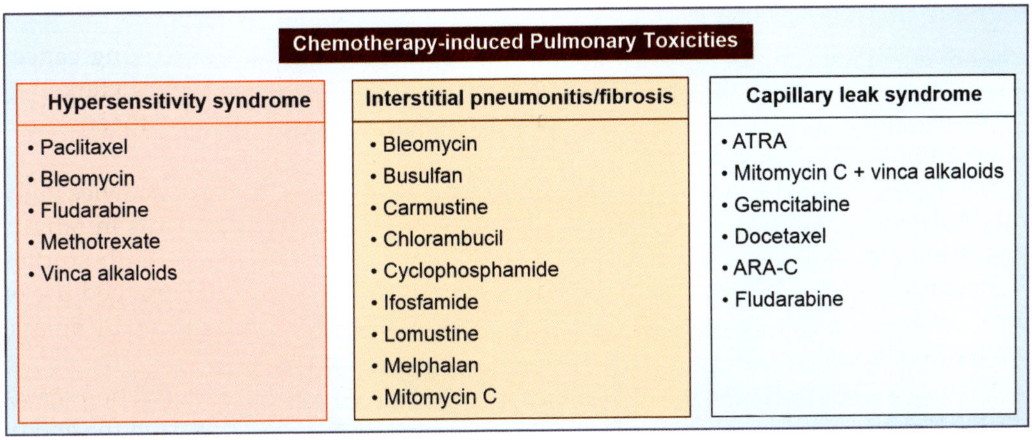

Fig. 12.2: Chemotherapy-induced pulmonary toxicities

toxicities can be broadly classified into three groups as depicted in Fig. 12.2. Although the optimal approach to dosing, timing, and duration of steroid use in these cases remains underexplored, the general practice involves administering around 0.5–1 mg/kg/day of prednisone or its equivalent for about 8–12 weeks.[16]

Taxanes: Docetaxel and paclitaxel, commonly used in non-small cell lung cancer (NSCLC) management, can trigger various pulmonary toxicities, predominantly presenting as interstitial lung disease-type symptoms. These reactions are often mediated by type IV T cell-mediated delayed hypersensitivity. Combining docetaxel with gemcitabine increases the risk of interstitial pneumonia. Imaging reveals diffuse ground-glass opacities (GGOs), and cases of non-specific interstitial pneumonitis and organizing pneumonia patterns have also been reported. Detecting other possible causes of respiratory distress such as infections is crucial, and treatment involves discontinuing taxols, administering high-dose steroids, and potentially using broad-spectrum antibiotics. While most patients recover, some may experience progressive respiratory failure.

Gemcitabine: Gemcitabine, commonly used and generally safe, can lead to pulmonary toxicities manifesting as worsening dyspnea, fever, chills, etc. Acute interstitial pneumonitis due to gemcitabine is thought to result from a cytokine-mediated hypersensitivity reaction, and the response to steroids can be variable.

Tyrosine Kinase Inhibitors (TKIs): The expanding array of TKIs used in lung cancer management has significantly improved outcomes. However, TKIs, particularly EGFR TKIs, can induce pulmonary toxicities like interstitial lung disease (ILD) or acute pneumonitis. Incidence rates vary globally, with the highest reported in Japan. Typically occurring within 4 weeks of treatment initiation, patients experience shortness of breath, hypoxia, cough, and fever. Inhibition of EGFR pathway-mediated repair processes underlies the development of interstitial pneumonitis.[17] Early radiological evaluation and exclusion of infections are crucial. Immediate cessation of the drug, followed by high-dose steroid initiation, is imperative due to the potentially high mortality associated with EGFR-TKI-associated ILD.

Immune-related Adverse Events

The advent of immunotherapy has significantly improved the outcomes of lung cancer patients. Among these immunotherapeutic agents, immune checkpoint inhibitors (ICPi) stand out, as they reinvigorate suppressed immune responses to combat cancer. However, this immune reinvigoration can sometimes disrupt immune homeostasis and trigger a distinct range of side effects known as immune-related adverse events (iRAEs). Unlike the typical side effects seen with chemotherapy or targeted therapy, iRAEs have their unique characteristics.

Corticosteroids remain the cornerstone in managing iRAEs. The treatment approach with steroids for iRAEs differs significantly from other medical indications. In this context, the duration and cumulative dose of steroids are often more extensive. Steroids are typically continued until the iRAEs resolve to grade 1 or better and are then gradually tapered over a span of 4–6 weeks.[18]

For managing iRAEs, several key strategies are employed. For grade 2 toxicities, it is often recommended to temporarily halt ICPis and resume treatment once symptoms or laboratory values revert to grade 1. Initial corticosteroid dosing typically starts at 0.5–1 mg/kg/day of prednisone or its equivalent.

When dealing with grade 3 toxicities, a more cautious approach is taken. ICP is typically paused, and high-dose corticosteroids are initiated, such as prednisone at a dosage of 1–2 mg/kg/day or its equivalent. If symptoms fail to improve within 48–72 hours of high-dose steroids, some cases might warrant the consideration of infliximab for certain toxicities.

Radiation Pneumonitis

Radiation pneumonitis is a consequence of the secondary effects of radiotherapy on lung tissue. The incidence of this condition is closely related to the volume of lung irradiated and the dose of radiation administered. It progresses through distinct phases: Acute, latent, exudative, intermediate, resolution, and fibrosis. Fibrosis, which predominantly manifests 6–8 months post-radiotherapy, continues to develop over time.[19]

Patients experiencing radiation pneumonitis often exhibit symptoms like non-productive cough, low-grade fever, and dyspnea. These symptoms typically appear 3–12 weeks post-treatment, but in some cases, they might even arise up to a year later. Chest CT scans are the preferred imaging method for diagnosing radiation pneumonitis.

Steroids are the primary agents employed in managing radiation pneumonitis.[20] For minimally symptomatic patients, a brief course of budesonide inhaler at 800 µg twice a day for 14 days is used. In cases of severe symptoms associated with subacute radiation pneumonitis, prednisone is administered (up to 60 mg/day) for 2–4 weeks, followed by a gradual tapering over 3–12 weeks.

However, once fibrosis sets in, the role of corticosteroids diminishes. At this stage, steroids no longer contribute to the management of radiation pneumonitis.

Allergic Reactions

Corticosteroids possess antiallergic properties, making them valuable in both preventing and treating drug infusion reactions, including severe cases like anaphylaxis and cytokine release or hypersensitivity reactions. Dexamethasone is the most commonly used agent in these scenarios.

In a proactive approach to managing hypersensitivity reactions, corticosteroids are often utilized alongside medications such as docetaxel, paclitaxel, etoposide, pemetrexed, amavantamab. This combination strategy aims to preemptively minimize the risk and severity of allergic or hypersensitivity responses to these drugs during infusion.

Chemotherapy-induced Nausea and Vomiting

Corticosteroids have a longstanding history as effective agents for preventing chemotherapy-induced nausea and vomiting (CINV). Moreover, they enhance the efficacy of other anti-emetic medications. Although the precise mechanisms underlying their actions in CINV prophylaxis and management are not fully understood, potential mechanisms include activating glucocorticoid receptors in the nucleus of the solitary tract and inhibiting and modulating 5HT-3A receptors.

In addressing acute CINV, corticosteroids are commonly combined with 5HT-3A antagonists, either alone or alongside NK1 inhibitors.[21] For highly emetogenic regimens, 24 mg of dexamethasone is administered when no NK1 antagonist is used, while 12 mg is given when used with an NK1 antagonist. In moderately emetogenic regimens, an 8 mg dose of dexamethasone is administered with a 5HT-3A antagonist.

For delayed CINV management, dexamethasone finds utility in both highly and moderately emetogenic chemotherapy regimens. Typical dosages in the delayed setting are 8 mg once or twice daily for 2–3 days.[22]

However, with the rise of chemotherapy and immunotherapy strategies for lung cancer, questions have emerged about the use of dexamethasone as a prophylactic anti-emetic agent.[23] This is due to the immunosuppressive properties of steroids. While specific data regarding dexamethasone-based CINV prophylaxis in the context of immunotherapy are scarce, extrapolation from other studies suggests that the use of dexamethasone preceding immune checkpoint inhibitor (ICI) treatment could potentially reduce its effectiveness.[24]

USE OF STEROIDS IN THE PATIENTS ON IMMUNOTHERAPY

The adverse effects of chemotherapy-induced nausea and vomiting (CINV) have raised significant concerns among patients undergoing chemotherapy. This has led to the utilization of dexamethasone alongside other medications to prevent CINV. However, due to the growing use of immune checkpoint inhibitors (ICIs) in conjunction with chemotherapy, there is a consideration about the simultaneous use of dexamethasone with ICIs. This raises the question of whether the immune-suppressing effects of dexamethasone could potentially diminish the effectiveness of ICIs.[23] The potential consequence of dexamethasone's immune-suppressing effects is that they might promote a state of immune tolerance towards tumours, thereby undermining the impact of ICIs. Research has shown that moderate increases in systemic glucocorticoids (GCs) can lead to the suppression of T cell activation signatures, causing the failure of treatments involving antiprogrammed death ligand-1 antibodies and CXCR4 antagonists in a model of genetically engineered pancreatic cancer. Given that tumors display unique antigens resulting from accumulated genetic alterations (neoantigens), it is conceivable that GC signaling might encourage immune tolerance towards tumors, ultimately diminishing the effectiveness of ICI treatments. It might be worth considering an alternative approach to dexamethasone-based prevention, focusing on using the smallest effective dose to alleviate symptoms. Existing guidelines from organizations like the National Comprehensive Cancer Network and the American Society of Clinical Oncology recommend a daily dose of 8–12 mg of dexamethasone on days 1–4 of each chemotherapy cycle. However, considering the prolonged effects of dexamethasone, it is probable that the heightened signaling of glucocorticoid receptors could persist for days or weeks after a 4-day dexamethasone regimen. Therefore, an alternative strategy that aims to use dexamethasone sparingly for prevention could potentially yield better results.

Adverse Events

The utilization of corticosteroids in various lung cancer management contexts, as discussed earlier, comes with several benefits. However, it is important to acknowledge that these agents can also lead to a range of potential adverse events (AEs), both during treatment and after discontinuation. These adverse events can be categorized into several groups (Fig. 12.3).

SITUATIONS REQUIRING PRUDENT STEROID USAGE

1. **Live vaccines:** Concurrent administration of live or live-attenuated vaccines should be avoided while on corticosteroid therapy, as these medications can potentially weaken the immune response to such vaccines.

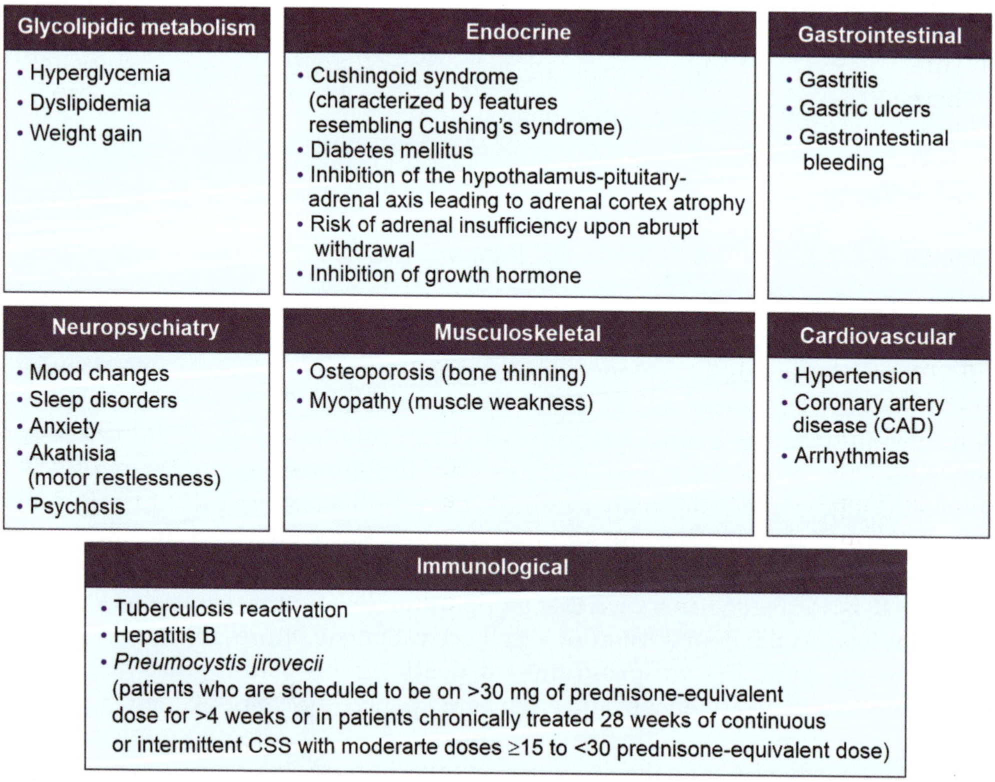

Fig. 12.3: Potential adverse events

2. **Diabetes:** Patients with diabetes mellitus need careful monitoring and management of blood glucose levels while on corticosteroids due to the potential to exacerbate hyperglycemia.
3. **Hypertension:** Individuals with poorly controlled arterial hypertension should be monitored closely, as corticosteroids can lead to an increase in blood pressure.
4. **Cardiovascular conditions:** Patients with heart failure, peripheral edema, or recent acute coronary syndrome need cautious corticosteroid usage, as these agents can have implications for cardiovascular health.
5. **Eye conditions:** Individuals with conditions like cataracts, glaucoma, or herpes simplex keratitis should exercise caution, as corticosteroids can worsen these eye conditions.
6. **GI health:** Those with a history of peptic ulcer disease may require careful corticosteroid use, as these agents can potentially aggravate gastrointestinal issues.
7. **Bone health:** Patients with low bone density, osteoporosis, or those at risk of bone collapse (e.g. due to bone metastases) should be monitored closely, as corticosteroids can contribute to bone loss.
8. **Liver function:** Individuals with liver disease should use corticosteroids with caution, as impaired liver function can affect drug metabolism.
9. **Psychiatric conditions:** Uncontrolled psychosis, behavioral problems, or alcohol dependence might be exacerbated by corticosteroid use, warranting careful consideration.
10. **Surgical healing:** Recent surgical interventions and wound healing issues require careful corticosteroid usage, as these agents can delay wound healing.
11. **Infections:** Active fungal, bacterial, or viral diseases (especially viral hepatitis, herpes, varicella, and shingles) can be worsened by corticosteroids due to their immunosuppressive effects.
12. **Epilepsy:** Individuals with uncontrolled or untreated epilepsy need cautious corticosteroid usage, as these agents can potentially interact with seizure medications.

Conclusion

As the field of lung cancer management continues to evolve, the role of steroids remains a subject of ongoing research and refinement. From addressing inflammation and enhancing treatment responses to mitigating adverse effects, their impact is undeniable. Steroids are crucial tools in addressing a range of challenges faced by lung cancer patients, from reducing chemotherapy-induced nausea and vomiting to managing radiation pneumonitis and immune-related adverse events. They serve as valuable components in the management of various symptoms, such as dyspnea and pain, contributing to improved quality of life.

In conclusion, the role of steroids in lung cancer management is multi-dimensional and pivotal. Recognizing their significance in various therapeutic scenarios while being vigilant about potential adverse effects ensures a holistic approach to patient care.

REFERENCES

1. Sung H, Ferlay J, Siegel RL, Laversanne M, Soerjomataram I, Jemal A, et al. Global Cancer Statistics 2020: GLOBOCAN Estimates of Incidence and Mortality Worldwide for 36 Cancers in 185 Countries. CA: *A Cancer Journal for Clinicians*. 2021;71(3):209–49.

2. Durham AL, Adcock IM. The relationship between COPD and lung cancer. Lung Cancer. 2015 Nov;90(2):121–7.
3. Ge F, Feng Y, Huo Z, Li C, Wang R, Wen Y, et al. Inhaled corticosteroids and risk of lung cancer among chronic obstructive pulmonary disease patients: a comprehensive analysis of nine prospective cohorts. Transl Lung Cancer Res. 2021 Mar;10(3):1266–76.
4. Schouten LJ, Rutten J, Huveneers HAM, Twijnstra A. Incidence of brain metastases in a cohort of patients with carcinoma of the breast, colon, kidney, and lung and melanoma. Cancer. 2002 May 15;94(10):2698–705.
5. Ryken TC, McDermott M, Robinson PD, Ammirati M, Andrews DW, Asher AL, et al. The role of steroids in the management of brain metastases: a systematic review and evidence-based clinical practice guideline. *J Neurooncol.* 2010 Jan;96(1):103–14.
6. Mulvenna P, Nankivell M, Barton R, Faivre-Finn C, Wilson P, McColl E, et al. Dexamethasone and supportive care with or without whole brain radiotherapy in treating patients with non-small cell lung cancer with brain metastases unsuitable for resection or stereotactic radiotherapy (QUARTZ): results from a phase 3, non-inferiority, randomised trial. The Lancet. 2016 Oct 22;388(10055):2004–14.
7. Kumar A, Weber MH, Gokaslan Z, Wolinsky JP, Schmidt M, Rhines L, et al. Metastatic Spinal Cord Compression and Steroid Treatment: A Systematic Review. Clin Spine Surg. 2017 May;30(4):156–63.
8. Campbell BA, Troupis JM, Langton J. Superior Vena Cava Obstruction. In: MacLeod RD, Van den Block L, editors. Textbook of Palliative Care [Internet]. Cham: Springer International Publishing; 2019 [cited 2023 Aug 27]. p. 1339–50. Available from: https://doi.org/10.1007/978-3-319-77740-5_73.
9. Leppert W, Buss T. The Role of Corticosteroids in the Treatment of Pain in Cancer Patients. Curr Pain Headache Rep. 2012;16(4):307–13.
10. Haywood A, Good P, Khan S, Leupp A, Jenkins-Marsh S, Rickett K, et al. Corticosteroids for the management of cancer-related pain in adults. Cochrane Database of Systematic Reviews [Internet]. 2015 [cited 2023 Aug 28];(4). Available from: https://www.cochranelibrary.com/cdsr/doi/10.1002/14651858.CD010756.pub2/full.
11. Laviano A, Meguid MM, Rossi-Fanelli F. Cancer anorexia: clinical implications, pathogenesis, and therapeutic strategies. The Lancet Oncology. 2003 Nov 1;4(11):686–94.
12. Roeland EJ, Bohlke K, Baracos VE, Bruera E, del Fabbro E, Dixon S, et al. Management of Cancer Cachexia: ASCO Guideline. JCO. 2020 Jul 20;38(21):2438–53.
13. Yavuzsen T, Davis MP, Walsh D, LeGrand S, Lagman R. Systematic Review of the Treatment of Cancer-Associated Anorexia and Weight Loss. JCO. 2005 Nov 20;23(33):8500–11.
14. Hui D, Bohlke K, Bao T, Campbell TC, Coyne PJ, Currow DC, et al. Management of Dyspnea in Advanced Cancer: ASCO Guideline. JCO. 2021 Apr 20;39(12):1389–411.
15. Lin RJ, Adelman RD, Mehta SS. Dyspnea in Palliative Care: Expanding the Role of Corticosteroids. J Palliat Med. 2012 Jul 1;15(7):834–7.
16. Delaunay M, Prévot G, Collot S, Guilleminault L, Didier A, Mazières J. Management of pulmonary toxicity associated with immune checkpoint inhibitors. European Respiratory Review [Internet]. 2019 Dec 31 [cited 2023 Aug 28];28(154). Available from: https://err.ersjournals.com/content/28/154/190012.
17. He Y, Zhou C. Tyrosine kinase inhibitors interstitial pneumonitis: diagnosis and management. Transl Lung Cancer Res. 2019 Nov;8(Suppl 3):S318–20.
18. Schneider BJ, Naidoo J, Santomasso BD, Lacchetti C, Adkins S, Anadkat M, et al. Management of Immune-related Adverse Events in Patients Treated with Immune Checkpoint Inhibitor Therapy: ASCO Guideline Update. JCO. 2021 Dec 20;39(36):4073–126.
19. Benveniste MF, Gomez D, Carter BW, Betancourt Cuellar SL, Shroff GS, Benveniste APA, et al. Recognizing Radiation Therapy-related Complications in the Chest. Radiographics. 2019 Mar;39(2):344–66.
20. Arroyo-Hernández M, Maldonado F, Lozano-Ruiz F, Muñoz-Montaño W, Nuñez-Baez M, Arrieta O. Radiation-induced lung injury: current evidence. BMC Pulmonary Medicine. 2021 Jan 6;21(1):9.

21. Hesketh PJ, Kris MG, Basch E, Bohlke K, Barbour SY, Clark-Snow RA, et al. Antiemetics: ASCO Guideline Update. JCO. 2020 Aug 20;38(24):2782–97.
22. Barbour SY. Corticosteroids in the Treatment of Chemotherapy-induced Nausea and Vomiting. *Journal of the National Comprehensive Cancer Network*. 2012 Apr 1;10(4):493–9.
23. Janowitz T, Kleeman S, Vonderheide RH. Reconsidering Dexamethasone for Antiemesis when Combining Chemotherapy and Immunotherapy. Oncologist. 2021 Apr;26(4):269–73.
24. Arbour KC, Mezquita L, Long N, Rizvi H, Auclin E, Ni A, et al. Impact of Baseline Steroids on Efficacy of Programmed Cell Death-1 and Programmed Death-Ligand 1 Blockade in Patients with Non-Small Cell Lung Cancer. JCO. 2018 Oct;36(28):2872–8.

Chapter

13

Steroids in Lung Transplantation and Complications

Chetan Vaddepally • Sri Charan

INTRODUCTION

Ever since the understanding of the role of the immune system in allograft dysfunction post-transplantation, corticosteroids were one of the initial groups of medications which were used to prevent allograft rejection post-transplantation. While the initial immunosuppressive strategies of total body radiation, combining it with azathioprine, 6-mercaptopurine proved futile, it was after the innovation of Dr. Thomas Starzl of adding prednisolone to azathioprine as maintenance immunosuppression that steroids were put in the forefront of immunosuppression.[1] Prof. James D. Hardy did the first human lung transplant in 1963 and used prednisolone along with azathioprine for maintenance immunosuppression.[2]

Solid organ transplants have been in vogue in India since 1971 when the first kidney transplant happened, and over the last 50 years, steroids have been the cornerstone of immunosuppression for solid organ transplants. The main reason for this is the role of steroids in all three signals of immunosuppression (Fig. 13.1).[3] Until recently, corticosteroids have been considered indispensable in immunosuppression strategies for solid organ transplants around the world.

MECHANISM OF ACTION OF STEROIDS

Glucocorticoids exert their anti-inflammatory and immunosuppressive effects by acting on the cytosolic glucocorticoid receptors (cGCRs). This GC-receptor complex translocates to the nucleus, where it activates the anti-inflammatory genes which is called transactivation. Glucocorticoids also cause repression of proinflammatory factors, which is called transrepression. While the immunosuppressive effects are mediated by both transactivation and transrepression, the adverse effects are mediated primarily by transactivation effects. In addition to this mechanism, in higher doses, i.e. pulsing doses, glucocorticoids exert what are known as non-genomic effects, which are mediated by membrane-bound GC receptors and ion channels about which less information is available. While the so-called genomic effects are cumulative dose-dependent and long-term, non-genomic effects are short-term and rapid onset in action.[4,5]

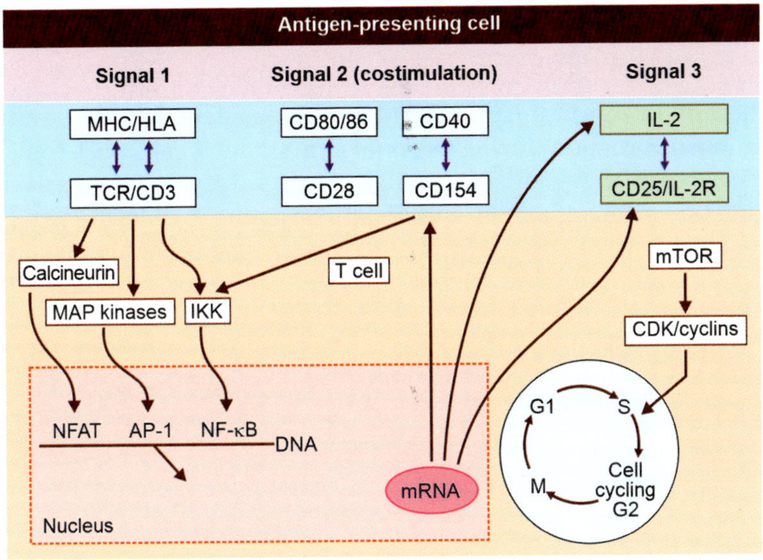

Fig. 13.1: The three-signal model of T-cell activation

MHC: Major histocompatibility complex; **HLA:** Human leukocyte antigens; **IL:** Interleukin; **TCR:** T cell receptor; **NFAT:** Nuclear factor of activated T cells; **mTOR:** Mammalian target of rapamycin

Glucocorticoids exert their immunosuppressive effects both on innate and adaptive immunity. The effects of glucocorticoids on various aspects of the immune system are summarized in Fig. 13.2.

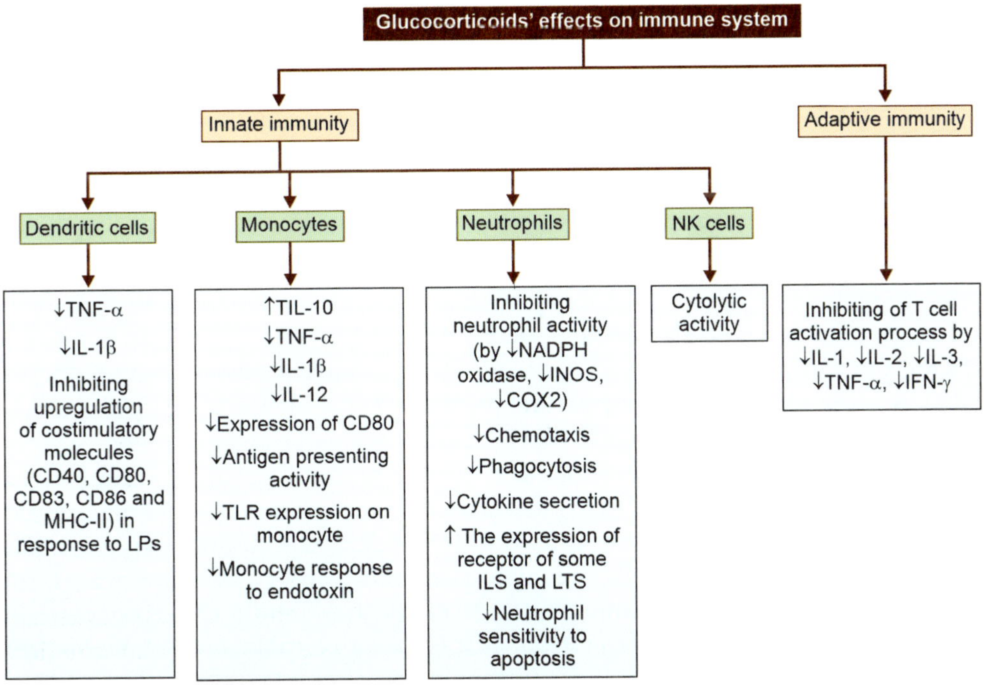

Fig. 13.2: Glucocorticoids' effects on immune system

STEROIDS IN LUNG TRANSPLANTATION

Induction Immunosuppression

Induction therapy in lung transplantation aims to achieve a potent and immediate state of immunosuppression during the crucial first few weeks post-transplant when acute rejection poses the greatest threat to graft survival. This early therapeutic window utilizes a variety of agents specifically targeting T cells, the key effector cells in rejection. This intensive short-term strategy employs potent agents like polyclonal and monoclonal T cell-depleting antibodies or IL-2 receptor antagonists (which both deplete T cell numbers and inhibit their activation) to rapidly mitigate the most critical rejection threats. By providing early protection, induction therapy paves the way for successful long-term graft survival and facilitates the transition to maintenance immunosuppression.[6,7]

ISHLT registry data reveals that exceeding 80% of lung transplant recipients receive induction therapy, encompassing polyclonal antilymphocyte preparations, anti-interleukin-2 receptor antibodies, and OKT3. Despite this widespread adoption, significant variability persists in the specific agent, dosage, and duration employed. This strategy rests on a threefold rationale:

1. Lung transplant recipients inherently face elevated rejection risk.
2. Induction therapy grants a safe window to achieve calcineurin inhibitor target levels without early rejection risk.
3. It allows renal recovery from surgical stress before calcineurin inhibitor exposure, thereby mitigating their potential nephrotoxicity.[7]

Though there are no clear-cut guidelines on the use of steroids as a part of induction immunosuppression, it is a common practice in all lung transplant programs across the world to give steroids intraoperatively. The dose of methylprednisolone given for induction varies from 1000 to 1500 mg at different centres. At our centre, we give intravenous methylprednisolone of 500 mg after intubation and 250 mg intravenous methylprednisolone before reperfusion of each lung, along with IL-2R antagonists like basiliximab. Similar protocols are followed in lung transplant centres worldwide.

Maintenance Immunosuppression

Lifelong immunosuppression remains the cornerstone of post-lung transplant care, aiming to prevent acute rejection, delay chronic allograft dysfunction, and ultimately improve patient survival. The era of modern maintenance regimens began in the 1990s with the introduction of modified cyclosporine, tacrolimus, and mycophenolic acid (MPA), leading to significant improvements in one-year allograft survival across all organ recipients by lowering rejection rates.[8]

Reflecting this shift, the 2019 Organ Procurement and Transplantation Network (OPTN) Annual Data Report (ADR) confirms a tacrolimus-mycophenolate mofetil (MMF)-corticosteroid combination as the dominant maintenance regimen (80%) for lung recipients, mirroring its prevalence in kidney (65%), pancreas (67%), liver (65%), and even heart (86%) transplants. Notably, tacrolimus and corticosteroids remain the preferred regimen for intestinal transplant recipients (44%), highlighting potential organ-specific considerations within the broader framework of maintenance immunosuppression (Fig. 13.3).

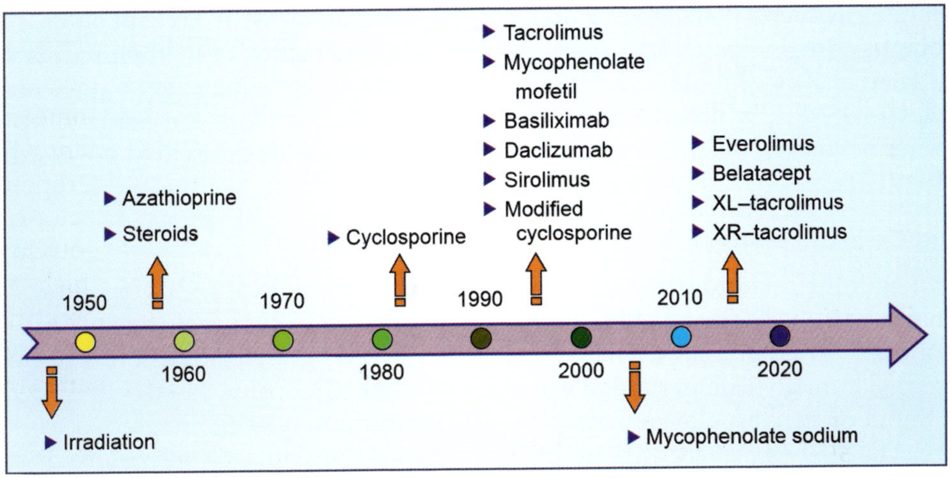

Fig. 13.3: Timeline of introduction of drugs for maintenance immunosuppression

Corticosteroids, along with azathioprine, remain one of the oldest-used immunosuppressant (Table 13.1) in any solid organ transplant. Intravenous methylprednisolone and oral prednisone are the most used corticosteroids for the prevention and treatment of rejection. All the patients who undergo lung transplantation shall be on lifelong corticosteroids. However, prolonged use of steroids is associated with significant morbidity. Hence, while withdrawal of steroids from maintenance immunosuppression has been attempted in other transplants, it is not recommended in lung transplant (Grade 2D recommendation),[9] but elimination efforts were made in 2 studies.

Borro et al withdrew steroids in 34 patients post-lung transplant and found that 80% remained off steroids.[10] Shirit et al withdrew steroids post-lung transplant in 35 patients, but it was associated with unstable PFTs and BOS in 21 patients, and they were continued back on steroids.[11] Our centre uses steroid methylprednisolone

Table 13.1: Most common immunosuppressant regimens at discharge[8]

Organ transplanted	*Regimen*
Kidney	Tacrolimus + MMF + corticosteroids (66%) Tacrolimus + MMF (27%)
Pancreas	Tacrolimus + MMF + corticosteroids (68%) Tacrolimus + MMF (26%)
Liver	Tacrolimus + MMF + corticosteroids (65%) Tacrolimus + MMF (17%) Tacrolimus + corticosteroids (6%)
Intestine	Tacrolimus + corticosteroids (37%) Tacrolimus + MMF + corticosteroids (30%) Tacrolimus + MMF (7%)
Heart	Tacrolimus + MMF + corticosteroids (86%) Tacrolimus + MMF (7%)
Lung	Tacrolimus + MMF + corticosteroids (82%) Other (11%)

IV initially, which is changed to oral prednisolone along with Mycophenolate and tacrolimus as maintenance immunosuppression. At our centre, IV methylprednisolone is initiated at 1 mg/kg/day, and it is tapered gradually by 5 mg every 5 days until it reaches 5 mg/day, which is continued lifelong. Similar protocols are used worldwide with minor changes like 250 mg/day of methylprednisolone in divided doses during the first 1–2 days.

Acute Cellular Rejection

Acute cellular rejection remains a significant threat in the first year after lung transplantation, with the ISHLT registry reporting a 28% incidence of treated episodes.[12,13] This pathology, a major contributor to early graft dysfunction, is primarily diagnosed through histological analysis of transbronchial biopsies. Based on the intensity and depth of perivascular mononuclear cell infiltration, rejection is graded from A0 (no rejection) to A4 (severe). Treatment typically involves pulsed corticosteroids, most commonly intravenous methylprednisolone 10–15 mg/kg daily or 500–1,000 mg daily for 3 days, followed by oral prednisolone tapering for A_2 and higher grades. However, optimal dosing and duration remain undefined by research. Notably, lymphocytic bronchiolitis, a distinct form of rejection, exhibits relative resistance to steroid therapy.[14] This lack of standardized optimal dosage and duration highlights the ongoing need for further research in this area.

Post-transplant Lymphoproliferative Disease

Post-transplant lymphoproliferative disease is a complication that occurs because of the reactivation of EBV post-transplant. While the treatment of PTLD is the withdrawal of immunosuppression, and chemotherapy, steroid (prednisolone) is used as a part of the chemotherapy regimen along with rituximab and CHOP.

DONOR MANAGEMENT

The proinflammatory cascade triggered by brain death significantly compromises the quality of donor lungs. To counter this detrimental effect and improve lung preservation, methylprednisolone administration has emerged as a crucial strategy in donor management. While routine steroid replacement is standard practice, studies highlight the efficacy of a specific high-dose regimen: 500 mg of methylprednisolone demonstrably increases lung acceptance rates. This targeted approach offers a promising avenue for optimizing lung quality and maximizing the potential for successful transplantation.[15]

COMPLICATIONS OF STEROID THERAPY IN LUNG TRANSPLANTATION

Infections: Glucocorticoids, while crucial for immunosuppression, are a double-edged sword, significantly increasing the risk of bacterial, fungal, and viral infections. The compromised immune system allows infections to disseminate, often with higher mortality. Fungal infections like mucormycosis, invasive aspergillosis, and *Pneumocystis jirovecii* pneumonia have become more potent threats. Notably, even moderate prednisolone doses (≥10 mg daily) raise the risk of respiratory viral infections like rhinovirus, coronavirus, and RSV, affecting roughly 25% of lung transplant recipients in the first year (Fig. 13.4).

Advantages	Disadvantages	Drug interactions
• Induction and maintenance of immunosuppression • Treatment of acute rejection • Treatment of recurrent autoimmune/inflammatory diseases after transplantation • Treatment of PTLD • Maintaining immunosuppression in patients with allograft loss and listed for retransplantation • Amelioration of IRI and maintaining donor lung quality	• Infections • Bone disorders • Growth retardation in children • Metabolic complications and cardiovascular risks • Neuropsychiatric side effects • Muscular side effects • Adrenal insufficiency • GI side effects • Other complications	• 3A4 inducers and inhibitors • CNIs

Fig. 13.4: Advantages and disadvantages of corticosteroids in lung transplantation

The long-term use of steroids further amplifies the risk of cytomegalovirus (CMV) infection and tuberculosis in post-transplant patients, necessitating careful monitoring and potentially adjusted immunosuppression strategies.

Obesity: Short-term glucocorticoid therapy is not associated with weight gain, but long-term glucocorticoid therapy is associated with weight gain. Steroids cause hyperplasia of adipose tissue, and they have anti-lipolytic effects. Steroids thus promote visceral obesity.[16,17]

Diabetes: Glucocorticoids cause hyperglycemia by causing insulin resistance. Risk factors for steroid-induced diabetes is obesity, history of diabetes in the family, history of gestational diabetes, and advanced age. The incidence of steroid-induced hyperglycemia is 32.3%, and steroid-induced diabetes is 18.6%. Weight control and diet management are important in controlling the incidence of steroid-induced hyperglycemia and diabetes.[18]

Lipid abnormalities: Steroids cause hypertriglyceridemia and hypercholesterolemia by inducing insulin resistance. Steroid increases the activity of acetyl-CoA carboxylase and fatty acid synthase, increases VLDL synthesis by the liver, and decreases the activity of lipoprotein lipase. Overall, it increases the levels of VLDL and LDL and decreases the levels of HDL.[19,20]

Hypercoagulability: Steroids cause thrombophilia, which, when coupled with obesity and decreased mobility, can predispose the patient to deep vein thrombosis.[21]

Cardiovascular disease: The cumulative effects of obesity, hypercoagulability, hypercholesterolemia, and insulin resistance predispose the patients to heart disease. Steroids also have a direct effect on the endothelial cells causing vascular dysfunction and atherogenesis.[22,23]

Neuropsychiatric complications: Long-term usage of steroids is also associated with increased anxiety, memory problems, sleep-related problems, and irritability. People with a history of psychiatric illnesses are at increased risk of these complications. They can also cause pseudotumor cerebri.

Bone-related complications: Steroids inhibit the differentiation of osteoblasts, they cause apoptosis of the osteoblasts, increase the effects of osteoclasts, and antagonize the effects of vitamin D. The net effect is that they cause bone resorption, osteoporosis, and increased risk of fractures.[24,25]

Muscles: Steroids have a direct effect on muscles. They decrease muscle protein synthesis and increase the rate of muscle catabolism. They are a risk factor in the development of myopathy, especially after large doses (pulse steroids).[26,27]

Growth in pediatric transplant recipients: Corticosteroids impair stature growth in children and prepubertal adolescents by inducing abnormal growth hormone secretion and response. Steroid-induced growth retardation in pediatric transplant patients encouraged SOT teams to apply steroid minimization protocols in prepubertal transplant patients with better bone health, growth outcome, and comparable allograft rejection rates.

Conclusion

Lung transplantation (LTx) has undergone a remarkable journey since the pioneering discovery of cyclosporine A (CSA) in the early 1980s. Subsequent breakthroughs in immunosuppressive drugs have ignited continuous hope for improving survival outcomes for lung transplant recipients. Corticosteroids remain the cornerstone of solid organ transplantation (SOT) due to their potent anti-inflammatory and immunosuppressive effects, particularly on the innate immune system. Additionally, glucocorticoid receptors (GRs) within the lung, liver, kidney, and heart offer significant tissue-protective mechanisms. However, adverse effects often manifest in non-target organs like bone, muscle, adipose tissue, the gastrointestinal tract, and skin.

Targeted delivery of glucocorticoids (GCs) using innovative approaches like nanoparticles or transporter-mediated prodrugs holds promise for maximizing efficacy and minimizing side effects in SOT. Directing GCs specifically to target organs like the liver, kidney, and heart could be a game-changer. Further research in this area is crucial for optimizing steroid therapy in transplant recipients.

Long-term triple-drug immunosuppression with tacrolimus (Tac), mycophenolate mofetil (MMF), and low-dose prednisone remains the standard of care for post-lung transplant patients. Deviations from this regimen are typically driven by individual patient intolerance and the need to manage unwanted side effects. While protocols vary between lung transplant centers, tailoring agent selection to each patient is essential. This individualized approach considers factors like time since transplant, rejection and infection history, side effect profile, and potential drug–drug interactions. Careful selection and vigilant monitoring of these high-risk medications are paramount to optimizing outcomes and ensuring longevity and improved quality of life for our patients.

REFERENCES

1. Barker CF, Markmann JF. Historical Overview of Transplantation. Cold Spring Harb Perspect Med. 2013 Apr 1;3(4): a014977–014977.
2. Hardy JD, Webb WR, Dalton ML, Walker GR. Special Contribution Lung Homotransplantation in Man Report of the Initial Case [Internet]. Available from: http://jama.jamanetwork.com.

3. Kumbala D, Zhang R. Essential concept of transplant immunology for clinical practice. *World J Transplant*. 2013;3(4):113.
4. Ponticelli C, Glassock RJ. Prevention of complications from use of conventional immunosuppressants: a critical review. *J Nephrol*. 2019 Dec 29;32(6):851–70.
5. Dashti-Khavidaki S, Saidi R, Lu H. Current status of glucocorticoid usage in solid organ transplantation. World J Transplant. 2021 Nov 18;11(11):443–65.
6. Small B, Au J, Brink H, Shah I, Strah H. Induction and maintenance immunosuppression in lung transplantation. *Indian Journal of Thoracic and Cardiovascular Surgery*. Springer; 2022;38:300–17.
7. Knoop C, Haverich A, Fischer S. Immunosuppressive therapy after human lung transplantation. *European Respiratory Journal*. 2004 Jan;23(1):159–71.
8. Nelson J, Alvey N, Bowman L, Schulte J, Segovia MC, McDermott J, et al. Consensus recommendations for use of maintenance immunosuppression in solid organ transplantation: Endorsed by the American College of Clinical Pharmacy, American Society of Transplantation, and the International Society for Heart and Lung Transplantation. Pharmacotherapy. 2022 Aug 1;42(8):599–633.
9. Nelson J, Alvey N, Bowman L, Schulte J, Segovia MC, McDermott J, et al. Consensus recommendations for use of maintenance immunosuppression in solid organ transplantation: Endorsed by the American College of Clinical Pharmacy, American Society of Transplantation, and the International Society for Heart and Lung Transplantation. Pharmacotherapy: *The Journal of Human Pharmacology and Drug Therapy*. 2022 Aug 29;42(8):599–633.
10. Borro JM, Solé A, De la Torre M, Pastor A, Tarazona V. Steroid Withdrawal in Lung Transplant Recipients. Transplant Proc. 2005 Nov;37(9):3991–3.
11. Shitrit D, Bendayan D, Sulkes J, Bar-Gil Shitrit A, Huerta M, Kramer MR. Successful steroid withdrawal in lung transplant recipients: result of a pilot study. Respir Med. 2005 May;99(5):596–601.
12. Chambers DC, Yusen RD, Cherikh WS, Goldfarb SB, Kucheryavaya AY, Khusch K, et al. The Registry of the International Society for Heart and Lung Transplantation: Thirty-fourth Adult Lung and Heart-Lung Transplantation Report—2017; Focus Theme: Allograft ischemic time. *Journal of Heart and Lung Transplantation*. 2017 Oct 1;36(10):1047–59.
13. Parulekar AD, Kao CC. Detection, classification, and management of rejection after lung transplantation. *J Thorac Dis*. 2019 Sep;11(S14): S1732–9.
14. Subramani MV, Pandit S, Gadre SK. Acute rejection and post-lung transplant surveillance. *Indian J Thorac Cardiovasc Surg*. 2022 Jul 22;38(S2):271–9.
15. Follette DM, Rudich SM, Babcock WD. Improved oxygenation and increased lung donor recovery with high-dose steroid administration after brain death. *J Heart and Lung Transplantation*. 1998 Apr;17(4):423–9.
16. Shen Y, Roh HC, Kumari M, Rosen ED. Adipocyte glucocorticoid receptor is important in lipolysis and insulin resistance due to exogenous steroids, but not insulin resistance caused by high fat feeding. Mol Metab. 2017 Oct;6(10):1150–60.
17. Kim HJ, Cha JY, Seok JW, Choi Y, Yoon BK, Choi H, et al. Dexras1 links glucocorticoids to insulin-like growth factor-1 signaling in adipogenesis. Sci Rep. 2016 Jun 27;6:28648.
18. Liu X xia, Zhu X ming, Miao Q, Ye H ying, Zhang Z yun, Li Y ming. Hyperglycemia Induced by Glucocorticoids in Nondiabetic Patients: A Meta-analysis. Ann Nutr Metab. 2014;65(4):324–32.
19. Sholter DE, Armstrong PW. Adverse effects of corticosteroids on the cardiovascular system. *Can J Cardiol*. 2000 Apr;16(4):505–11.
20. Meng X, Chen X, Wu L, Zheng S. The Hyperlipidemia Caused by Overuse of Glucocorticoid after Liver Transplantation and the Immune Adjustment Strategy. *J Immunol Res*. 2017;2017:1–5.
21. Coelho MCA, Santos CV, Vieira Neto L, Gadelha MR. Adverse effects of glucocorticoids: coagulopathy. *Eur J Endocrinol*. 2015 Oct;173(4):M11-21.
22. Anagnostis P, Athyros VG, Tziomalos K, Karagiannis A, Mikhailidis DP. Clinical review: The pathogenetic role of cortisol in the metabolic syndrome: a hypothesis. *J Clin Endocrinol Metab*. 2009 Aug;94(8):2692–701.
23. Walker BR. Glucocorticoids and cardiovascular disease. *Eur J Endocrinol*. 2007 Nov;157(5):545–59.

24. Frenkel B, White W, Tuckermann J. Glucocorticoid-induced Osteoporosis. Adv Exp Med Biol. 2015; 872:179–215.
25. Buckley L, Humphrey MB. Glucocorticoid-induced Osteoporosis. *N Engl J Med*. 2018 Dec 27;379(26):2547–56.
26. Khaleeli AA, Edwards RH, Gohil K, McPhail G, Rennie MJ, Round J, et al. Corticosteroid myopathy: a clinical and pathological study. Clin Endocrinol (Oxf). 1983 Feb;18(2):155–66.
27. Pereira RMR, Freire de Carvalho J. Glucocorticoid-induced myopathy. Joint Bone Spine. 2011 Jan;78(1):41–4.

Chapter

14

Tapering of Steroids in Lung Diseases

Dutta Reddy

INTRODUCTION

Glucocorticoids (GCs) are frequently used in clinical practice because of their potent anti-inflammatory and immunosuppressive effects. The prevalence of GC use in India is around 1.8%.[1] Exogenous steroid intake can cause adrenal gland atrophy and secondary adrenal insufficiency. Steroids in any form, like systemic, topical, inhaled, ocular, intra-nasal, and intra-articular, can cause hypothalamic-pituitary-adrenal (HPA) axis suppression. There is a significant inter-individual variability in steroid response. The suppression of the HPA axis may continue even after GC withdrawal, which leads to adrenal insufficiency. HPA suppression is a serious medical concern, which can cause an acute adrenal crisis that is potentially life-threatening if unidentified and treated timely. If the patient received chronic steroid therapy, the steroids should be tapered gradually, and HPA axis evaluation should be done before withdrawing the steroids.

PHARMACOLOGY OF GLUCOCORTICOIDS

Steroids have various effects on most of the cells through the action at the level of the nucleus. They modulate the immune function and cause various metabolic effects. Systemic steroids can be classified into short-acting (hydrocortisone), intermediate-acting (prednisolone, methylprednisolone), and long-acting (dexamethasone), depending on their duration of action. In lung diseases, steroids are usually used systemically, like intravenous, oral, or inhalational routes.

Pharmacological doses of steroids are used to treat various inflammatory (Table 14.1), allergic, and immunological diseases; if used for prolonged periods (>2–3 weeks), they cause various adverse effects, importantly adrenal suppression.[2]

Table 14.1: Steroid equivalent doses

Steroid	*Equivalent dose*
Hydrocortisone	20 mg
Deflazacort	6 mg
Prednisolone	5 mg
Methylprednisolone	4 mg
Triamcinolone	4 mg
Dexamethasone	0.75 mg
Betamethasone	0.75 mg

GLUCOCORTICOID-INDUCED ADRENAL INSUFFICIENCY

The hypothalamic-pituitary-adrenal axis controls the endogenous secretion of cortisol. Cortisol, in turn, inhibits the ACTH release from the pituitary through negative feedback control (Fig. 14.1). Exogenous steroids similarly suppress the ACTH release from the pituitary gland. GC-induced adrenal insufficiency (AI) should be suspected in patients who took more than 30 mg of hydrocortisone per day orally (bioequivalent doses of prednisolone >7.5 mg, dexamethasone >0.75 mg) for more than 3 weeks. Along with the dose of the steroid, the timing of the steroid also affects the HPA suppression (a higher evening dose of steroid suppresses ACTH more than a higher morning dose). The prevalence of steroid-induced AI depends on the dose, duration, route of administration, and type of steroid. A systematic review by Rebecca et al found the median prevalence of steroid-induced AI is 37.4%.[3]

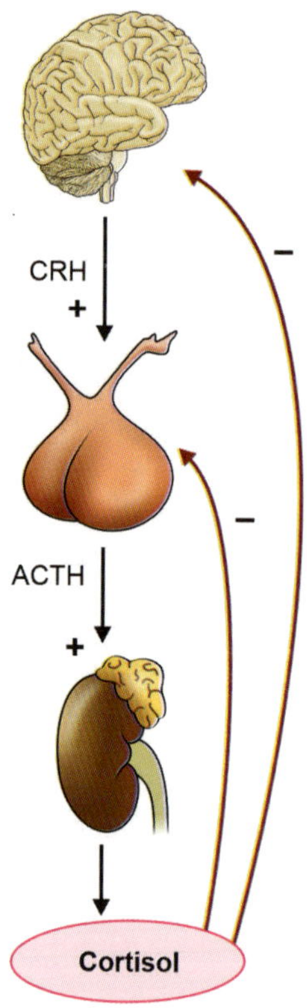

Fig. 14.1: Hypothalamic-pituitary-adrenal (HPA) axis

WITHDRAWAL OF GLUCOCORTICOIDS

If the underlying lung disease permits withdrawal of steroids, steroids should be reduced from pharmacological doses to physiological doses (reduce the dose rapidly, like 2.5 mg of prednisolone every 3–4 days) to 7.5 mg of prednisolone per day over a few weeks. After that dose should be reduced by 1 mg of prednisolone every 2–4 weeks, depending on the patient's tolerability. A different approach is to convert 5 mg of prednisolone to 20 mg of hydrocortisone and then reduce the hydrocortisone dose 2.5 mg every week till 10 mg per day of hydrocortisone. Then maintain a stable dose of 10 mg per day of hydrocortisone for 2 to 3 months. After that, the endogenous function of the HPA axis is assessed by basal 8 AM serum cortisol levels. If the basal cortisol is more than 14.5 µg/dl, it indicates an intact HPA axis and the steroid is safely withdrawn. If the basal cortisol is less than 3 µg/dl, it is highly suggestive of secondary adrenal insufficiency. Steroids should be continued till the recovery of the HPA axis. If cortisol values are in between, dynamic testing is required. The insulin tolerance test is the gold standard test, but it is cumbersome and rarely done. ACTH stimulation test (short synacthen test—SST) is a good alternative dynamic test. In SST, 250 µg of synthetic ACTH (tetracosactrin) is injected intravenous or intramuscular, and plasma cortisol is measured at 30 and 60 minutes. If the cortisol is more than 14–16 µg/dl, depending on the assay, it indicates recovery of the HPA axis, then the steroid can be withdrawn safely (Table 14.2).

Table 14.2: Steroid withdrawal plan

Dose of steroid (equivalent of prednisolone)	*Duration of steroid treatment*	*Duration of steroid treatment*
	≤3 weeks	**>3 weeks**
≥7.5 mg/day	Can stop	Reduce the dose rapidly, like 2.5 mg of prednisolone every 3–4 days
		↓
5–7.5 mg	Can stop	Reduce 1 mg every 2–4 weeks
		↓
<5 mg	Can stop	Reduce 1 mg every 2–4 weeks (or) convert 5 mg of prednisolone to 20 mg of hydrocortisone (HC), then reduce HC 2.5 mg weekly till 10 mg per day of HC, after 2–3 months test for HPA axis recovery

REFERENCES

1. Rachel Mulavelil, et al. Glucocorticoid use and misuse in a rural community of Kerala, India. *Indian J Endocrinol Metab*. 2022 May-Jun; 26(3):234–238.
2. Dennis M Williams. Clinical Pharmacology of Corticosteroids. Respir Care 2018;63(6):655–670.
3. Rebecca M Joseph, et al. Systemic glucocorticoid therapy and adrenal insufficiency in adults: A systematic review. J. Semarthrit. 2016;03:001.

Chapter

15

Adverse Effects of Steroids

G Uma Sri • M Ramakrishna Reddy

INTRODUCTION

While corticosteroids are invaluable for their potent anti-inflammatory effects, their long-standing use carries a shadow of potential side effects. These adverse effects, ranging from mild to life-threatening, depend heavily on the dose and duration of therapy, often manifesting as a single issue or a complex interplay of multiple ones. Notably, these side effects are the primary reason why corticosteroid use is often limited. It is usually at "supra-physiological" doses that glucocorticoids unleash a cascade of adverse effects, ranging from significant suppression of the hypothalamic-pituitary axis to severe, life-threatening infections.

The underlying molecular mechanisms for GC-mediated adverse effects are complex and only partly understood. Some glucocorticoid-induced adverse effects, like diabetes and glaucoma, are primarily driven by transactivation, while others, such as suppression of the hypothalamic-pituitary-adrenal (HPA) axis, are more reliant on transrepression.[1] Beyond dose and duration, several other factors influence the severity of these side effects, including age, underlying health conditions, and nutritional status.[2] Therefore, careful monitoring and dose optimization are crucial when using corticosteroids to maximize their therapeutic benefit while minimizing the risk of associated risks.

MUSCULOSKELETAL ADVERSE EFFECTS

Glucocorticoid-induced Osteoporosis

For patients receiving chronic oral glucocorticoid therapy, vigilant monitoring of bone mineral density (BMD) is crucial. Up to 40% of these individuals develop bone loss, increasing fracture risk.[3] This accelerated bone loss arises from a multifactorial interplay: Enhanced osteoclast activity via RANK-ligand upregulation, diminished osteoblast and osteocyte function and number, and ultimately, impaired bone formation alongside accelerated resorption.[3] This imbalance between osteogenesis and osteolysis favors rapid bone deterioration, with trabecular bone bearing the initial brunt (within 6–12 months) and cortical bone succumbing with prolonged use. Notably, osteoporotic fractures, particularly vertebral, have been documented even in patients with average BMD.[4] Therefore, preventive measures with bisphosphonates or estrogen therapy in postmenopausal women may be warranted when BMD levels approach the borderline or low range.

Steroid-induced Myopathy

Chronic corticosteroid therapy carries the risk of reversible, painless muscle weakness, known as steroid-induced myopathy. This non-inflammatory myopathy directly stems from muscle breakdown and affects both upper and lower limbs, primarily the proximal muscles. Unlike inflammatory myopathies, muscle enzymes like creatine kinase and aldolase remain within normal limits, and electromyography findings lack specificity. Muscle biopsy, however, reveals atrophy of fast-twitch type II fibers without any signs of inflammation.[5] Fortunately, discontinuing corticosteroid use and engaging in appropriate exercises typically lead to the resolution of steroid-induced myopathy.

Osteonecrosis

Prolonged glucocorticoid use (prednisolone 20 mg) daily carries the dreaded risk of avascular necrosis (AVN), particularly affecting the femoral head. This serious complication manifests initially as pain, which can progressively intensify and limit daily activities. Early detection is crucial, and magnetic resonance imaging (MRI) is the gold standard for its high sensitivity. Conservative management prioritizes reduced weight-bearing and immobilization. In the early stages, where osteonecrosis might be reversible, and the weight-bearing portion is spared, core decompression surgery can be considered. The core decompression, combined with concentrated bone marrow containing mesenchymal stem cells, can offer significant pain relief, improve function, and even halt AVN progression.[6] However, when the joint damage becomes irreversible and progresses to osteoarthritis, total joint replacement becomes the only viable option.

DERMATOLOGIC ADVERSE EFFECTS

While topical corticosteroids offer potent relief for inflammatory skin conditions, long-term use can come with a spectrum of dermatologic side effects. These include easy bruising, skin thinning, steroid-induced acne and facial redness, striae, impaired wound healing, hair loss, and perioral dermatitis. Corticosteroids inhibit protein synthesis, leading to decreased collagen production, which manifests as thin, easily bruised skin (dermal atrophy).[7] Additionally, the increased fragility of blood vessels within the thinned skin further contributes to the development of purpura, characterized by small red or purple dots. Striae, often seen as stretch marks, arise when the skin overstretches, causing internal vessels to rupture. A study by Karagas and colleagues suggests a potential link between long-term topical steroid use and an increased risk of non-melanoma skin cancer, specifically SCC (squamous cell carcinoma).[8]

METABOLIC AND ENDOCRINE ADVERSE EFFECTS

Diabetes Mellitus

Chronic systemic glucocorticoid use poses a significant threat to blood sugar control, leading to a dose-dependent increase in both fasting and postprandial sugar levels, even in individuals without pre-existing diabetes. This prolonged hyperglycemia is not merely an inconvenience but a potential trigger for the development of both diabetes mellitus and central obesity, which in turn further exacerbates insulin resistance, creating a vicious cycle.[9]

Cushingoid Features

Prolonged exposure to high-dose systemic corticosteroid, exceeding physiological levels, carries a characteristic side effect profile termed "Cushingoid features." These distinctive characteristics include truncal obesity (fat accumulation around the trunk), a prominent "buffalo hump" between the shoulders, a rounded face known as "moon facies," and overall weight gain (Fig. 15.1). Notably, the frequency of these features

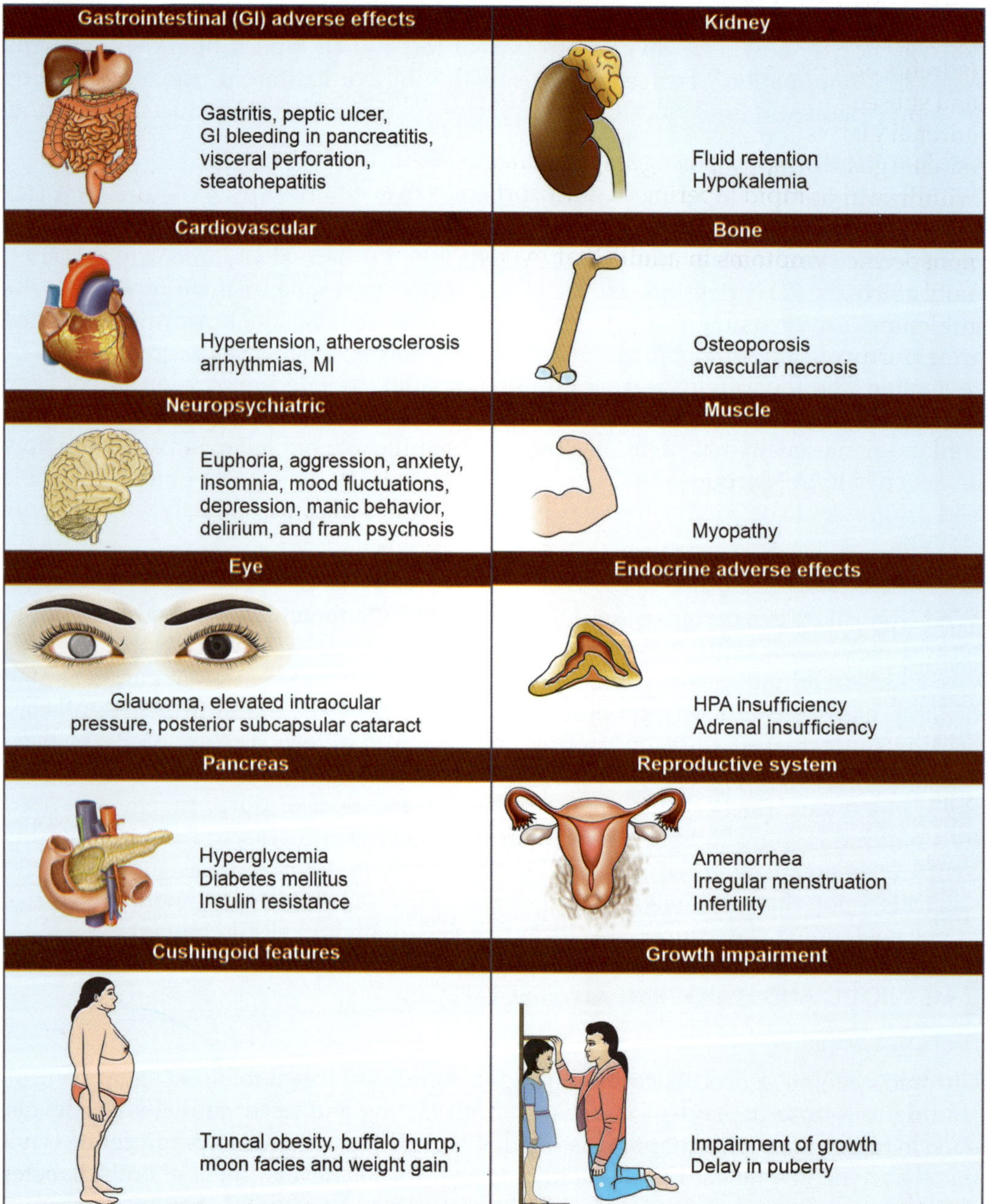

Fig. 15.1: Adverse effects of steroids

exhibits a linear correlation with the dose and duration of corticosteroid therapy, underscores the importance of careful monitoring and dose optimization during chronic corticosteroid therapy.[10]

Suppression of HPA Axis

Prolonged glucocorticoid therapy directly suppresses the hypothalamic-pituitary-adrenal (HPA) axis by inhibiting CRH (corticotropin-releasing hormone) production from the hypothalamus, leading to decreased ACTH (adrenocorticotropic hormone) release from the pituitary and subsequently, diminished cortisol production by the adrenal glands (Fig. 15.2). ACTH deficiency can lead to adrenal gland atrophy, posing a significant threat. Abrupt withdrawal or rapid tapering of glucocorticoids in such patients can trigger an adrenal crisis characterized by nonspecific symptoms in adults that may go unnoticed until a stressor like illness, surgery, or injury overwhelms the compromised adrenal glands. Therefore, careful monitoring of HPA axis function and gradual dose reduction are crucial to mitigate this risk and ensure safe glucocorticoid use.

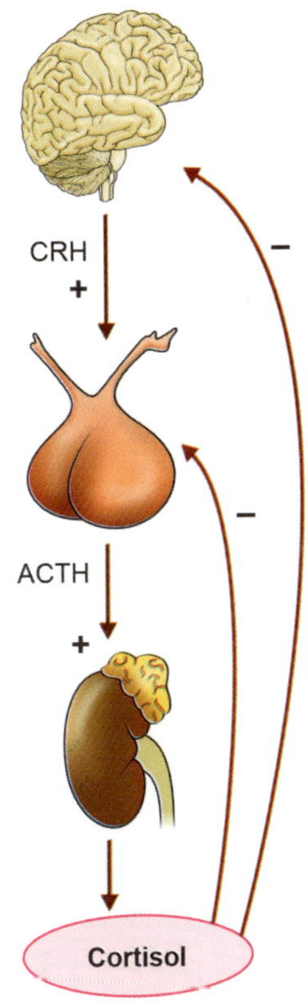

Fig. 15.2: Hypothalamic-pituitary-adrenal axis

GROWTH IMPAIRMENT

Young children receiving long-term glucocorticoids, especially daily oral steroids or high-dose inhaled forms, experience growth impairment and delayed puberty. This effect is most common in chronic illnesses like asthma or nephrotic syndrome. While daily steroids carry the biggest risk, even inhaled corticosteroids can impact growth at higher doses due to their systemic absorption and cortisol suppression. Importantly, growth impairment in this context can be an independent adverse effect of the medication itself, or it can be a sign of underlying adrenal suppression caused by steroid therapy.[11] In prepubertal children, this initial decrease in height can persist into adulthood, with an average reduction of around 1 cm in final height. Therefore, careful monitoring of growth and timely dose adjustments are crucial for minimizing this potential risk and ensuring optimal health outcomes in young patients reliant on glucocorticoids.

CARDIOVASCULAR ADVERSE EFFECTS

Prolonged hyperglycemia induced by glucocorticoids (GCs) sets the stage for a cascade of cardiovascular risks. By promoting insulin resistance and hyperinsulinemia, GCs trigger increased production of very low-density lipoproteins (VLDLs) and triglycerides, fueling fat storage and dyslipidemia. Additionally, GCs directly activate enzymes involved in fatty acid synthesis and decrease lipoprotein lipase activity, further elevating VLDL and LDL levels while lowering protective HDL.[12] Some GCs exert weak mineralocorticoid effects, leading to edema, weight gain, and electrolyte imbalances (like hypokalemia and metabolic alkalosis), contributing to potential arrhythmias. These metabolic and hemodynamic alterations ultimately accelerate atherosclerosis, increasing the risk of significant cardiovascular complications such as coronary artery disease, stroke, and heart failure.[13] A recent population study by Wei et al highlights this concern, suggesting that supraphysiological GC doses may be associated with higher rates of these cardiovascular events and even all-cause mortality. Therefore, careful consideration of cardiovascular risks and close monitoring are crucial when administering GCs, especially in high doses and for prolonged periods.

GASTROINTESTINAL (GI) ADVERSE EFFECTS

Prolonged glucocorticoid use increases the risk of adverse GI effects, including gastritis, gastric ulcer formation, and GI bleeding. Healing of existing peptic ulcers can also be impaired. Additionally, complications like pancreatitis, visceral perforation, and even fatty liver can occur. Combining glucocorticoids with NSAIDs further multiplies the risk of GI complications by fourfold.[14] Therefore, proton pump inhibitors are often recommended for patients taking both medications, especially at high doses or for prolonged periods.

NEUROPSYCHIATRIC ADVERSE EFFECTS

Glucocorticoid therapy carries a risk of various neuropsychiatric disturbances, ranging from euphoria, aggression, anxiety, and insomnia to more complex manifestations like mood swings, depression, manic behavior, delirium, and even frank psychosis. While these disturbances often resolve with time after stopping the medication, a concerning minority of patients may experience persistent symptoms. Therefore, careful monitoring and dose optimization are needed to mitigate these potential risks.[15]

INFECTIONS

Prolonged glucocorticoid use weakens the immune system, increasing the risk of both common and life-threatening infections. This vulnerability often goes unnoticed as glucocorticoids dampen the body's inflammatory response, masking typical signs and symptoms of infection, making early diagnosis challenging. While elevated neutrophil count is seen with these medications, it does not reflect true immune improvement but rather a mobilization of existing white blood cells. The risk extends to bacterial, fungal, and viral infections, with immunocompromised patients often experiencing more severe and disseminated forms, leading to significantly higher mortality. Notably, glucocorticoid therapy significantly increases the risk of fungal infections like mucormycosis, invasive aspergillosis, and *Pneumocystis jirovecii* pneumonia, highlighting the need for careful monitoring and proactive infection prevention strategies.[16]

OPHTHALMOLOGIC ADVERSE EFFECTS

Long-term glucocorticoid therapy leads to various ophthalmologic adverse effects, most commonly posterior subcapsular cataracts affecting both eyes with gradual progression. Another potential risk is steroid-induced glaucoma, often presenting painlessly but carrying the threat of irreversible visual field loss, optic nerve excavation, and damage. Additionally, a rarer complication is central serous chorioretinopathy, characterized by blurred central vision and reduced visual acuity. Early detection and timely management are crucial to minimize the impact of these potential risks associated with prolonged glucocorticoid use.[17]

REPRODUCTIVE SYSTEM ADVERSE EFFECTS

Prolonged corticosteroid therapy can impact the reproductive system in both men and women. In women, this may manifest as menstrual irregularities or amenorrhea, while in men, it can lead to decreased sperm production and motility. Additionally, pregnant women receiving corticosteroids face the risk of fetal intrauterine growth retardation, highlighting the need for careful monitoring and dose optimization during pregnancy.[18,19]

SIDE EFFECTS OF INHALATIONAL CORTICOSTEROIDS

Examining the fate of an inhaled corticosteroid (ICS) is crucial to understanding its safety profile. Figure 15.3 offers a schematic representation of this complex journey. Upon inhalation, a significant portion deposits in the mouth and pharynx, posing a risk for local side effects like thrush or irritation. If not rinsed away, this portion can be swallowed and potentially absorbed in the gut, contributing to systemic exposure. Furthermore, any drug escaping inactivation by first-pass metabolism in the liver enters the bloodstream directly, potentially leading to extrapulmonary side effects.[20]

While the portion reaching the lungs delivers the desired anti-inflammatory action, a substantial amount can be absorbed back into the systemic circulation via the pulmonary vasculature, again contributing to potential systemic side effects (Table 15.1). Therefore, understanding the pharmacokinetic properties of an ICS, such as its deposition pattern,

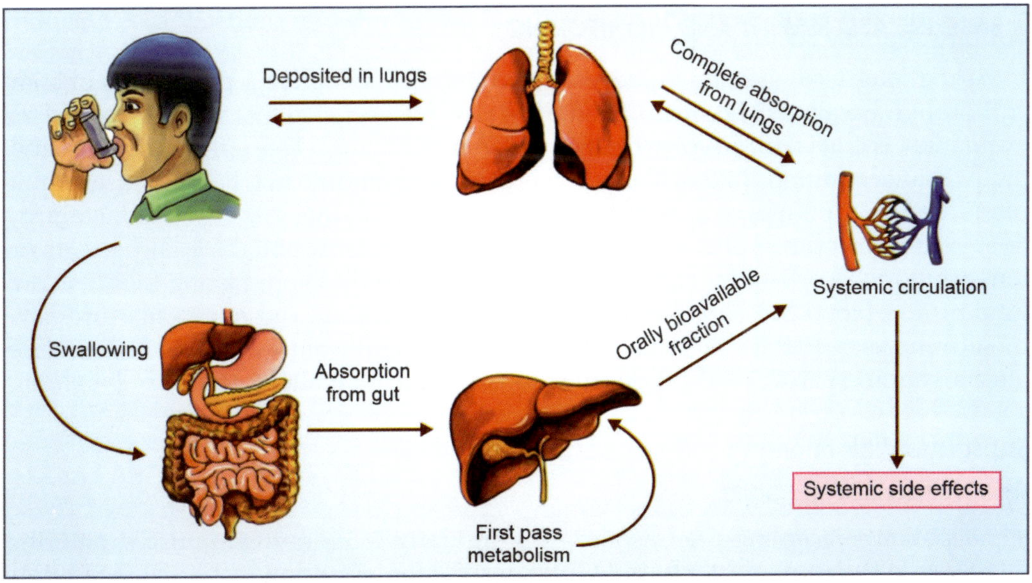

Fig. 15.3: Fate of inhalational corticosteroids

Table 15.1: Potential local and systemic side effects of inhaled corticosteroids[20]

Local side effects	*Systemic side effects*
• Bronchospasm	• Adrenal crisis
• Dysphonia	• Growth impairment
• Oropharyngeal candidiasis	• Skin thinning
• Pharyngitis	• Skin bruising
• Reflex cough	• Cataract and glaucoma
• Sore throat	• Osteoporosis and bone fractures

oral bioavailability, and pulmonary absorption, is vital for predicting its safety profile. This knowledge, coupled with understanding the pharmacodynamic characteristics, like receptor affinity and duration of action, allows clinicians to carefully balance the intended benefits with potential risks when choosing the right ICS for each patient. The most common local oropharyngeal adverse effects of inhaled corticosteroids are oral candidiasis, dysphonia, and hoarseness of voice. The use of a spacer device or Aero-Chamber significantly reduces these side effects.

CONTRAINDICATIONS TO USE OF SYSTEMIC CORTICOSTEROIDS

1. Hypersensitivity to any component of the formulation.
2. Concurrent administration of live or live-attenuated vaccines.
3. Systemic fungal infection, herpes simplex keratitis, and varicella infection.
4. Osteoporosis and low bone mineral density.
5. Uncontrolled diabetes mellitus and hypertension.
6. Glaucoma.

BASELINE ASSESSMENT AND MONITORING

Initiating long-term systemic glucocorticoid therapy demands a prudent approach. A thorough baseline assessment, including a comprehensive history and risk factor evaluation, is crucial to optimize treatment and minimize adverse effects. Patients with pre-existing conditions like diabetes, hypertension, dyslipidemia, heart failure, peptic ulcers, and osteoporosis require careful monitoring due to their increased vulnerability to steroid-induced complications. Regular monitoring is essential for all patients on long-term glucocorticoids. This includes pl ysical examination, fasting blood sugar, lipid profile, blood pressure measurement, weight tracking, and intraocular pressure monitoring, is crucial for these patients. In cases of significant steroid-related adverse effects, steroid-sparing medications may be explored as an alternative.[21]

Subsequent Monitoring for Glucocorticoid Therapy[22]

Assessment of Bone Health

- All patients receiving prednisone ≥2.5 mg daily ≥3 months require promoting adequate calcium and vitamin D intake, smoking cessation, eat a balanced diet, engage in regular weight-bearing exercise, and limiting alcohol intake.

- DEXA scan: Ideally, before/within 6 months of therapy initiation for adults ≥40 or those <40 with risk factors.
- 10-year fracture risk assessment using the FRAX tool for adults ≥40.
- Lateral spine X-ray for ≥65 years to assess vertebral fractures.
- Treatment based on fracture risk category:
  - **<40 years:** Bisphosphonates/teriparatide/denosumab for moderate/high risk.
  - **≥40 years:** Bisphosphonates/teriparatide/denosumab/raloxifene for moderate/high risk.

HPA Axis Function

- Assess if systemic corticosteroids are used >2 consecutive weeks, >3 cumulative weeks in the past 6 months, or with persistent adrenal suppression symptoms.
- Screen with early morning salivary cortisol after dose tapering.
- Perform low-dose ACTH stimulation test for persistent symptoms despite normal cortisol.
- Consider endocrinology referral for confirmation.

Growth in Children/Adolescents

Monitor growth every 6 months and plot on a growth curve.

Dyslipidemia and Cardiovascular Risk (Adults)

- Monitor lipid profile 1 month after initiation and every 6–12 months thereafter.
- Monitor glycemic control: Screen for classic symptoms (polyuria, polydipsia, weight loss) at every visit. Check glucose parameters for 48 hours after initiation, then every 3–6 months for 1 year, then annually. Consider annual oral glucose tolerance test for obese children with diabetes risk factors.

Ophthalmological Complications

- Consider annual ophthalmologic examination, especially for cataract symptoms.
- Refer for intraocular pressure assessment if there is a personal/family history of glaucoma, diabetes, or high myopia.

This comprehensive monitoring approach ensures timely identification and management of potential complications associated with long-term glucocorticoid therapy, improving patient outcomes.

Prevention of Adverse Effects

While some adverse effects of glucocorticoids are inevitable, several strategies can help minimize their occurrence:

1. **Dose optimization:** Employing the lowest effective dose for the shortest duration is paramount to achieving treatment goals while reducing risk.
2. **Comorbidity management:** Addressing pre-existing conditions like diabetes or hypertension can mitigate the impact of glucocorticoids on these systems.
3. **Patient monitoring:** Regular monitoring for potential adverse effects, including opportunistic infections and bone loss, allows for timely intervention.
4. **Concomitant medication management:** Patients on NSAIDs or anticoagulants require concomitant proton pump inhibitor (PPI) therapy to prevent peptic ulcers. While the

consensus on PPI use for patients on glucocorticoids alone is lacking, individual risk factors should be considered.

5. **Immunization:** Appropriate vaccinations are crucial before initiating long-term or high-dose glucocorticoid therapy.
6. ***Pneumocystis jirovecii* pneumonia (PCP) prophylaxis:** Patients receiving prednisone ≥20 mg daily for ≥2 weeks require prophylaxis against PCP, discontinuing once the dose falls below 20 mg.
7. **Infection assessment:** Carefully assess for active or potential infections, as glucocorticoids are generally contraindicated in such scenarios.
8. **Drug interaction awareness:** Be mindful of potential interactions between glucocorticoids and other medications being used concomitantly.

By implementing these strategies, healthcare professionals can significantly reduce the risk of adverse effects associated with glucocorticoid therapy, ensuring optimal patient outcomes.

REFERENCES

1. Schäcke H, Döcke WD, Asadullah K. Mechanisms involved in the side effects of glucocorticoids. Pharmacol Ther. 2002 Oct;96(1):23-43. doi: 10.1016/s0163-7258(02)00297-8. PMID: 12441176.
2. Huscher D, Thiele K, Gromnica-Ihle E, Hein G, Demary W, Dreher R, Zink A, Buttgereit F. Dose-related patterns of glucocorticoid-induced side effects. Ann Rheum Dis. 2009 Jul;68(7):1119–24.
3. Dykman TR, Gluck OS, Murphy WA, Hahn TJ, Hahn BH. Evaluation of factors associated with glucocorticoid-induced osteopenia in patients with rheumatic diseases. Arthritis Rheum. 1985 Apr;28(4):361–8.
4. Weinstein RS. Glucocorticoid-induced osteonecrosis. Endocrine. 2012;41(2):183–90.
5. Schakman O, Gilson H, Thissen JP. Mechanisms of glucocorticoid-induced myopathy. *Journal of Endocrinology*. 2008;197(1):1–10.
6. Houdek MT, Wyles CC, Martin JR, Sierra RJ. Stem cell treatment for avascular necrosis of the femoral head: current perspectives. Stem Cells Cloning. 2014 Apr 9;7:65-70. doi: 10.2147/SCCAA.S36584. PMID: 24744611; PMCID: PMC3986287.
7. Schoepe S, Schäcke H, May E, Asadullah K. Glucocorticoid therapy-induced skin atrophy. Experimental Dermatology. 2006;15(6):406–20.
8. Karagas MR, Cushing Jr GL, Greenberg ER, Mott LA, Spencer SK, Nierenberg DW. Non-melanoma skin cancers and glucocorticoid therapy. *British Journal of Cancer*. 2001;85(5):683–86.
9. Garrapa GG, Pantanetti P, Arnaldi G, Mantero F, Faloia E. Body composition and metabolic features in women with adrenal incidentaloma or Cushing's syndrome. The Journal of Clinical Endocrinology and Metabolism. 2001;86(11):5301–6.
10. Arnaldi G, Angeli A, Atkinson AB, Bertagna X, Cavagnini F, Chrousos GP, Fava GA, Findling JW, Gaillard RC, Grossman AB, Kola B. Diagnosis and complications of Cushing's syndrome: A consensus statement. *The Journal of Clinical Endocrinology and Metabolism*. 2003;88(12):5593–5602.
11. Lai HC, FitzSimmons SC, Allen DB, Kosorok MR, Rosenstein BJ, Campbell PW, Farrell PM. Risk of persistent growth impairment after alternate-day prednisone treatment in children with cystic fibrosis. *New England Journal of Medicine*. 2000;342(12):851–9.
12. Wei L, MacDonald TM, Walker BR. Taking glucocorticoids by prescription is associated with subsequent cardiovascular disease, Ann Intern Med, 2004, vol. 141.
13. Souverein PC, Berard A, Van Staa TP, Cooper C, Egberts AC, Leufkens HG, Walker BR. Use of oral glucocorticoids and risk of cardiovascular and cerebrovascular disease in a population-based case–control study. Heart. 2004;90(8):859–65.

14. Rodríguez LA, Hernández-Díaz S. The risk of upper gastrointestinal complications associated with nonsteroidal anti-inflammatory drugs, glucocorticoids, acetaminophen, and combinations of these agents. Arthritis Research and Therapy. 2000;3(2):98–101.
15. Keenan PA, Jacobson MW, Soleymani RM, Mayes MD, Yaldoo DT. The effect on memory of chronic prednisone treatment in patients with systemic disease. Neurology. 1996;47(6):1396–402.
16. Auphan N, DiDonato JA, Rosette C, Helmberg A, Karin M. Immunosuppression by glucocorticoids: Inhibition of NF-κB activity through induction of I κB synthesis. Science. 1995;270(5234):286.
17. Carvalho-Recchia CA, Yannuzzi LA, Negrão S, Spaide RF, Freund KB, Rodriguez Coleman H, Lenharo M, Iida T. Corticosteroids and central serous chorioretinopathy. Ophthalmology. 2002;109(10): 1834–7.
18. Whirledge S, Cidlowski JA. Glucocorticoids, stress, and fertility. Minerva Endocrinologica. 2010;35(2):109–1.
19. Sugden MC, Langdown ML, Munns MJ, Holness MJ. Maternal glucocorticoid treatment modulates placental leptin and leptin receptor expression and materno-fetal leptin physiology during late pregnancy, and elicits hypertension associated with hyperleptinaemia in the early-growth-retarded adult offspring. *European Journal of Endocrinology*. 2001;145(4):529–39.
20. Derendorf H, Nave R, Drollmann A, Cerasoli F, W. Relevance of pharmacokinetics and pharmacodynamics of inhaled corticosteroids to asthma. *Wurst European Respiratory Journal* Nov 2006;28(5):1042–1050; DOI: 10.1183/09031936.00074905.
21. Janahi IA, Rehman A, Baloch NUA. Corticosteroids and their use in Respiratory Disorders [Internet]. Corticosteroids. InTech; 2018. Available from: http://dx.doi.org/10.5772/intechopen.72147.
22. Yasir M, Goyal A, Sonthalia S. Corticosteroid Adverse Effects. [Updated 2023 Jul 3]. In: StatPearls [Internet]. Treasure Island (FL): StatPearls Publishing; 2024 Jan-. Available from: https://www.ncbi.nlm.nih.gov/books/NBK531462.

Chapter

16

Steroids in Miscellaneous Lung Diseases

M Ramakrishna Reddy • G Uma Sri

CORTICOSTEROIDS IN PLEURAL DISEASES

Steroids for Pleural Infection

Any pleural effusion secondary to community-acquired pneumonia (bacterial, viral) is called parapneumonic effusion and is associated with intense pleural inflammation. These effusions are characterized by elevated levels of proinflammatory cytokines, including interleukin-6 (IL-6), interleukin-8 (IL-8), tumor necrosis factor-α (TNF-α), vascular endothelial growth factor (VEGF), and monocyte chemotactic protein (MCP).[1] The early intervention aimed at modulating the inflammatory cascade may hold promise in preventing fibrinolytic dysregulation and subsequent loculations, ultimately facilitating pleural fluid drainage.[2]

The steroid therapy and outcome of parapneumonic pleural effusions (STOPPE) trial, a landmark multicenter, double-blinded, randomized controlled trial, investigated the potential of targeting the inflammatory response in parapneumonic effusions with corticosteroids to improve clinical outcomes. Patients with community-acquired pneumonia and associated pleural effusion were randomized to receive intravenous dexamethasone 4 mg twice daily for 48 hours or placebo and followed for 30 days. Ultimately, the STOPPE trial demonstrated that corticosteroid administration did not offer significant clinical benefit in these patients, challenging the notion of early anti-inflammatory intervention as a universally effective strategy for managing parapneumonic effusions.[3]

Steroids in TB Pleural Effusion

Pleural tuberculosis (TB) remains a significant cause of exudative pleural effusions, particularly in tuberculosis-endemic settings and among HIV-positive individuals. Its pathogenesis hinges on a delayed-type (type IV) hypersensitivity reaction elicited by the release of mycobacterial antigens into the pleural cavity. These antigens typically originate from the rupture of a subpleural focus of pulmonary TB infection.

The rationale for corticosteroid use in pleural TB rests on its ability to dampen the exuberant type IV hypersensitivity response triggered by released mycobacterial antigens. This response is considered the driver of tuberculous pleurisy, with its characteristic constellation of fever, progressive pleural effusion, and malaise. Theoretically, suppressing this inflammatory cascade could ameliorate these clinical manifestations.

The efficacy of adjunctive corticosteroids in treating tuberculous pleural effusion remains a topic of debate. A recent Cochrane meta-analysis by Ryan et al, encompassing 6 trials with 590 participants, investigated their potential benefits. The analysis suggested that corticosteroids may expedite pleural effusion resolution and minimize the risk of chronic pleural thickening and adhesions. However, data regarding their impact on post-treatment respiratory function remains inconclusive. Notably, corticosteroid use carries an increased risk of adverse events necessitating treatment discontinuation. Epigastric pain, hypertension, and hyperglycemia are frequently reported side effects.

Given the very low mortality associated with pleural tuberculosis and the lack of robust evidence demonstrating significant improvements in long-term respiratory function, corticosteroids are not recommended for the treatment of pleural tuberculosis. Current guidelines do not recommend the use of corticosteroids in pleural TB.[4,5]

REACTIVE AIRWAY DYSFUNCTION SYNDROME

Reactive airway dysfunction syndrome (RADS) is an acute, asthma-like illness characterized by the sudden onset of respiratory symptoms following high-level exposure to irritant gases, fumes, or vapors in the respiratory tract.

Diagnostic Criteria

- Documented absence of pre-existing respiratory disease.
- Confirmed exposure to an irritant gas, smoke, fume, or vapor in high concentration.
- Symptoms develop within 24 hours of exposure and persist for at least 3 months.
- Asthma-like symptoms: Cough, wheezing, shortness of breath.
- Pulmonary function tests may show airway obstruction.

Management

Current evidence lacks well-defined guidelines for managing RADS, either acutely or long-term. Most individuals experiencing short-term exposure to the offending agent recover spontaneously without significant clinical or radiological sequelae. As airway inflammation forms the initial pathogenic basis, the use of high-dose oral corticosteroids in symptomatic patients following acute exposure remains a logical therapeutic approach, although further research is warranted.[6]

LARYNGOTRACHEITIS (CROUP)

Croup, a frequent cause of upper airway obstruction in children, typically arises from infection with the parainfluenza virus (predominantly type 1). Characterized by hoarseness, barking cough, and inspiratory stridor, it primarily affects children under 3 years of age, with boys slightly more susceptible.

Despite its self-limiting nature, croup's frequent emergency visits and hospitalizations strain healthcare systems significantly. The culprit lies in localized inflammation of the subglottic region, the narrowest part of the upper airway. This edema significantly increases airway resistance, leading to difficult breathing in young children. In some cases, inflammation can rarely extend to the lower airways, culminating in laryngotracheobronchitis or even, rarely, superimposed bacterial laryngotracheobronchopneumonitis.[7]

Croup management prioritizes relieving symptoms and diminishing inflammation through multifaceted approaches. Glucocorticoids form the cornerstone of therapy. Supportive care, including humidified oxygen therapy, proper hydration, and antipyretics, lays the foundation. In addition to supportive care and corticosteroids, nebulized epinephrine may be used in severe cases with significant airway obstruction. Studies, including a meta-analysis by Kairys et al, have shown significant clinical improvement and reduced intubation rates within 12 hours of steroid administration compared to placebo. While the current standard oral dexamethasone dose is 0.6 mg/kg, research suggests this may be higher than necessary for optimal efficacy.[8]

CYSTIC FIBROSIS

Cystic fibrosis (CF), an autosomal recessive disorder, arises from mutations in the CFTR gene, leading to impaired chloride transport in epithelial cells. This dysfunction manifests primarily in the airways and is characterized by chronic mucus build-up, recurrent pulmonary infections, and progressive lung damage. Inhalation of *Aspergillus conidia*, particularly common in CF due to compromised mucociliary clearance, can establish lung colonization. In susceptible individuals, this colonization can trigger an immune response and inflammatory cascade, leading to allergic bronchopulmonary aspergillosis (ABPA) and further complicating the respiratory course of CF.

Corticosteroid use in cystic fibrosis (CF) management remains a point of debate. Randomized controlled trials indicate that routine use in non-asthmatic, non-ABPA patients offers little benefit and potential harm. However, short-term systemic therapy shows promise during acute infective exacerbations.[9] A study by Tepper et al[10]' showed significant and sustained improvements in lung function when a short course of intravenous hydrocortisone was added to standard treatment in patients with an acute infective exacerbation of CF.[10]

TRACHEAL HEMANGIOMA

Despite being the most prevalent benign vascular tumors in children, hemangiomas rarely involve the trachea and, to an even lesser extent, the larynx, posing a unique clinical challenge due to their uncommon location and potential impact on the airway. Clinically, patients with tracheal hemangiomas often experience characteristic symptoms like stridor, respiratory distress, progressive dyspnea, chronic cough, and even hemoptysis. Bronchoscopy remains the mainstay of diagnosis, providing direct visualization of the lesion and aiding in tissue collection for biopsy.

While less definitive, imaging techniques like CT scans and MRI can offer valuable insights into the extent and involvement of surrounding structures. Treatment for tracheal hemangiomas requires a tailored approach based on the severity and characteristics of the lesion. Propranolol may be considered for smaller lesions and mild symptoms, local steroid injections for localized control, systemic steroids for extensive lesions, and surgical resection as a last resort for severe cases with life-threatening airway obstruction.[11]

REFERENCES

1. Komissarov AA, Rahman N, Lee YCG, Florova G, Shetty S, Idell R, et al. Fibrin turnover and pleural organization: bench to bedside. *Am J Physiol Lung Cell Mol Physiol* 2018;314:L757–L768.
2. Arnold DT, Maskell NA. Corticosteroids for Pleural Infection: Should We STOPPE Studying? *Am J Respir Crit Care Med.* 2022 May 1;205(9):987-988. doi 10.1164/rccm.202201-0057ED. PMID: 35139316; PMCID: PMC9851490.
3. Fitzgerald DB, Waterer GW, Budgeon C, Shrestha R, Fysh ET, Muruganandan S, et al. Steroid Therapy and Outcome of Parapneumonic Pleural Effusions (STOPPE): a pilot randomized clinical trial. *Am J Respir Crit Care Med* 2022;205:1093–101.
4. Ryan H, Yoo J, Darsini P. Corticosteroids for tuberculous pleurisy. Cochrane Database Syst Rev. 2017 Mar 14;3(3):CD001876. doi: 10.1002/14651858.CD001876.pub3. PMID: 28290161; PMCID: PMC5461868.
5. Ryan H, Yoo J, Darsini P. Corticosteroids for tuberculous pleurisy. Cochrane Database Syst Rev [Internet]. 2017 [cited 2019 Sep 8];(3). Available from: https://www.cochranelibrary.com/cdsr/doi/10.1002/14651858.CD001876.pub3/ful.
6. Alberts WM, do Pico GA. Reactive airways dysfunction syndrome. Chest. 1996; 109:1618–26.
7. Cherry JD. Clinical practice. Croup. *New England Journal of Medicine*. 2008;358(4):384–91.
8. Brown JC. The management of croup. Br Med Bull. 2002; 61:189–202. doi: 10.1093/bmb/61.1.189. PMID: 11997306.
9. Balfour-Lynn IM, Welch K. Inhaled corticosteroids for cystic fibrosis. Cochrane Database of Systematic Reviews. 2016;8:CD00191.
10. Tepper RS, Eigen H, Stevens J, Angelicchio C, Kisling J, Ambrosius W, Heilman D. Lower respiratory illness in infants and young children with cystic fibrosis. Pediatric Pulmonology. 1997;24(1):48–51.
11. Buckmiller L, Dyamenahalli U, Richter GT. Propranolol for airway hemangiomas: case report of novel treatment. Laryngoscope 2009; 119:2051–2054.

Chapter

17

Guideline Recommendations for Steroids in Lung Diseases

G Uma Sri • M Ramakrishna Reddy

COMMUNITY-ACQUIRED PNEUMONIA (CAP)

Current guidelines for corticosteroid use in CAP are cautious. The 2019 IDSA/ATS guidelines advise against routine use in both mild and severe cases, including influenza pneumonia. However, they support using corticosteroids in severe CAP patients with septic shock unresponsive to other treatments, aligning with Surviving Sepsis Campaign recommendations. Decisions for patients in intensive care remain complex. The 2017 South African guidelines suggest considering corticosteroids (e.g. methylprednisolone 0.5 mg/kg every 12 hours) for severe CAP unless influenza, tuberculosis, or recent gastrointestinal bleeding is suspected (Table 17.1). The more recent 2023 ERS/ESICM/ESCMID/ALAT guidelines recommend corticosteroids for severe CAP patients with shock, excluding those with viral causes (influenza, SARS, MERS), uncontrolled diabetes, or ongoing corticosteroid use for other reasons. Methylprednisolone (0.5 mg/kg every 12 hours for 5 days) is a potential option in these specific severe CAP cases.

Table 17.1: Current guideline recommendations for corticosteroid use in CAP[1]

Guideline	*Drug*	*Dose*	*Duration*	*Year*
ATS/IDSA[2]	Do not use	–	–	2019
BTS	Do not use	–	–	2009
SEPAR[3]	Not specified	–	–	2010
South African[4]	Methylprednisolone	0.5 mg/kg/12 hour	5 days	2017
ERS/ESICM/ESCMID/ALAT[5]	Methylprednisolone	0.5 mg/kg/12 hour	5 days	2023

COVID-19 PNEUMONIA

Current guidelines from WHO/ERS/NIH (2020), IDSA (2022), and NICE (2023) recommend dexamethasone 6 mg daily for 7–10 days as the standard corticosteroid treatment for hospitalized COVID-19 patients requiring supplemental oxygen (Table 17.2). This medication can be administered orally or intravenously. If dexamethasone is unavailable, alternative corticosteroids with equivalent anti-inflammatory effects may

Table 17.2: Current guideline for corticosteroid use in COVID-19 pneumonia[1]

Guideline (reference)	*Preferred drug*	*Daily dose (mg)*	*Duration (days)*	*Degree of recommendation*	*Year*
EMA[6]	Dexamethasone	6	Up to 10	Strong	2020
WHO[7]	Dexamethasone	6	Up to 10	Conditional	2020
IDSA[8]	Dexamethasone	6	10 or until hospital discharge	Strong	2022
ERS[9]	Dexamethasone	6	Up to 10	Strong	2020
NIH[10]	Dexamethasone	6	10 or until hospital discharge	Strong	2020

be considered, such as prednisone (40 mg daily), methylprednisolone (32 mg daily), or hydrocortisone (160 mg daily).

ASTHMA

The Global Initiative for Asthma (GINA) guidelines recommend a tailored approach to corticosteroid use in asthma, depending on severity. For mild asthma (steps 1 and 2), a low-dose inhaled corticosteroid (ICS) combined with formoterol used only when needed (as-needed ICS–formoterol) is preferred to minimize unnecessary medication use while ensuring quick symptom relief. Alternative options include daily low-dose ICS or combining an ICS with each use of a short-acting β-agonist (SABA) inhaler. In moderate asthma (steps 3 and 4), single-inhaler maintenance and reliever therapy (SMART) with a low- or medium-dose ICS–formoterol combination becomes the mainstay for both ongoing control and rapid symptom relief. Alternative options involve either low- or medium-dose ICS–LABA with as-needed SABA or as-needed ICS–SABA combination inhalers. For severe asthma (step 5), GINA emphasizes personalized therapy based on specific characteristics. While high-dose ICS remains a cornerstone, additional controller medications or frequent oral corticosteroids may be needed. Biologics like omalizumab or mepolizumab can be targeted towards specific inflammatory markers like high IgE or eosinophils, potentially reducing reliance on high-dose ICS and oral steroids. GINA guidelines recommend a short course of oral corticosteroids (OCS) to manage asthma exacerbations, but not for routine use. For adults, the typical dose is prednisolone 40–50 mg daily for 5–7 days (Table 17.3). Children aged 6–11 years receive a slightly lower dose based on weight (1–2 mg/kg/day, maximum 40 mg/day) for 3–5 days. Importantly, tapering these medications is generally not advised in asthma

Table 17.3: Current guideline for corticosteroid use in asthma[1]

Guideline (reference)	*Drug*	*Dose (mg)*	*Duration*	*Year*
GINA[11]	Prednisone	40–50	5 to 7 days	2023
ATS[12]	Prednisone	37.5–50	7 days	2019
BTS[13]	Prednisone	40–50	5–7 days	2019
Swiss[14]	Prednisone	40–50	Up to 7 days	2018
NAEPP[15]	Prednisone	40	Up to 7 days	2020
Japan[16]	Prednisolone	0.5 mg/kg body weight	Usually less than 7 days	2020
TSANZ[17]	Prednisone	40	5–10 days	2021

exacerbations, but prompt administration within the first hour of an exacerbation is essential for optimal effectiveness.

CHRONIC OBSTRUCTIVE PULMONARY DISEASE (COPD)

While inhaled corticosteroids (ICS) offer limited benefits for most COPD patients due to distinct inflammatory pathways compared to asthma, they can be useful for those with an overlapping asthma component (ACOS) and elevated eosinophils. Conversely, for moderate-to-severe COPD exacerbations, short-course oral corticosteroids (prednisolone or equivalent) are the mainstay treatment, improving symptoms and lung function and reducing hospital stays. However, their use requires careful consideration of individual characteristics, exacerbation severity, and potential side effects. International guidelines consistently recommend them, with a standard regimen of 40 mg prednisolone equivalent daily for 5 days (Table 17.4). The ERS/ATS task force suggests a conditional recommendation for a slightly longer course (≤14 days) for outpatients with potential benefits in lung function and hospitalization reduction, but limited data on mortality and adverse effects necessitates further research for stronger endorsement. Importantly, prolonged courses of corticosteroids should be avoided due to increased pneumonia and mortality risks. The optimal timing for initiating corticosteroids in COPD exacerbations remains unclear, but earlier administration is likely beneficial. While TSANZ guidelines recommend tapering for extended courses (>14 days), the lack of significant recurrence difference in studies without tapering suggests abrupt withdrawal might be acceptable. Further research is needed to definitively determine the best approach for corticosteroid initiation and withdrawal timing in COPD exacerbations.

Table 17.4: Current guideline for corticosteroid use in COPD[1]

Guideline	*Drug*	*Daily dose (mg)*	*Duration (days)*	*Year*
GOLD[19]	Prednisolone	40	5	2023
ATS/ERS[20]	Prednisone	30–40	10–14	2017
NICE[21]	Prednisolone	30	5	2019
Can Thor Soc[22]	Prednisone or equivalent	30–50	5–10	2010
Japan[23]	Prednisolone	30–40	7–10	2019
TSANZ[24]	Prednisolone	30–40	5	2019

ACUTE RESPIRATORY DISTRESS SYNDROME (ARDS)

The efficacy of corticosteroids in ARDS remains a topic of ongoing research and debate, with various studies reporting conflicting outcomes. These discrepancies likely stem from a multitude of methodological factors, including variations in study design, underlying etiology of ARDS, corticosteroid dosage, initiation timing, treatment duration, specific tapering strategies, and the type of corticosteroid employed. Reflecting this evolving understanding, guidelines cautiously endorse corticosteroids. The 2017 SCCM/ESICM guidelines cautiously recommend corticosteroids for ARDS patients with a PaO_2/FiO_2 ratio below 200. More recently, JRS/JSICM/JSRCM-GL2021 and FICM/ICS-GL 2018 guidelines offer weak to strong recommendations based on specific scenarios (Table 17.5). While the optimal type and dose of steroids remain

Table 17.5: Current guideline for corticosteroid use in ARDS[1]

Guideline (reference)	*Indication*	*Drug*	*Daily dose*	*Duration*	*Tapering*	*Degree of recommendation*
SCCM/ ESICM[25]	Moderate-to-severe ARDS	Methylprednisolone	1 mg/kg	14 days	Yes, over 14 days	Conditional
BTS/ICM/ ICSGDG[26]	Mild-to-severe ARDS	Not specified	–	–	–	Further research
JPCG[27]	Not specified	Methylprednisolone	1–2 mg/kg	At least 7 days	Not specified	Conditional
SRLF[28]	Moderate-to-severe ARDS	Methylprednisolone	1 mg/kg	14 daysa	Yes	Conditional

under investigation, research suggests that low-dose administration (approximately 1–2 mg/kg methylprednisolone equivalent) initiated early in the disease course and continued for at least seven days may be beneficial. The DEXA-ARDS trial confirmed reduced ventilation duration and improved 60-day mortality with early administration of dexamethasone. Importantly, prolonged high doses should be avoided due to potential complications, and corticosteroids should be tapered gradually (6–14 days) to prevent rebound inflammation.

SEPSIS

Current guidelines for corticosteroid use in septic shock are cautious, recommending them only as an adjunct therapy after adequate fluid resuscitation and vasopressors fail to improve the condition. While the overall safety and efficacy of corticosteroids remain under debate due to study heterogeneity, evidence suggests they may shorten the duration of shock, ventilator use, and ICU stay. If used, cortisol at a dose of 200 mg/day continuously or 60 mg bolus four times daily is recommended for at least 3 days, and can typically be discontinued after vasopressor cessation. Notably, there is no clear consensus on tapering or abrupt withdrawal, as larger trials without tapering showed no difference in shock recurrence.

ALLERGIC BRONCHOPULMONARY ASPERGILLOSIS (ABPA)

The International Society for Human and Animal Mycology (ISHAM-ABPA) developed diagnostic guidelines for ABPA in 2013.[29] Recognizing advancements in the field, they recently published revised clinical practice guidelines (Agarwal et al, 2024) that encompass diagnosis, classification, and treatment of allergic bronchopulmonary aspergillosis/mycoses.[30] Prednisolone remains a mainstay in treating acute ABPA flare-ups, but the ideal dosage remains a topic of discussion. Traditionally, regimens like Greenberger (2002), with a starting dose of 0.5 mg/kg daily for 2 weeks followed by a tapering schedule aimed for discontinuation around 3 months, were commonly used.[31] However, some patients require longer-term, low-dose maintenance corticosteroids to prevent relapse. On the other hand, some physicians favor a more aggressive approach, like the high-dose regimen proposed by Agarwal et al (2008), starting with 0.75 mg/kg daily for 6 weeks, transitioning to a lower dose for another 6 weeks, and potentially extending treatment with a maintenance dose for up to a year.[32,33] Recognizing this variability, recent ISHAM-ABPA guidelines (2024) acknowledge the effectiveness of both high and low-dose prednisolone for controlling exacerbations. However, they highlight the advantage of lower doses (around 0.5 mg/kg/day for 2–4 weeks) with fewer side effects, even if the initial response might be slower. To address this, some centers have adopted intermediate tapering regimens with doses like 0.5 mg/kg, 0.25 mg/kg, and 0.125 mg/kg daily for four weeks each, then tapered by 5 mg every two weeks till discontinuation (Table 17.6). This approach seeks to balance effectiveness with minimizing side effects.[30]

Initial therapy for acute ABPA typically involves a low-to-moderate dose of oral prednisolone (0.5 mg/kg/day for 2–4 weeks) tapered over four months.[30] Oral itraconazole for four months serves as an alternative for patients where systemic glucocorticoids are contraindicated. Notably, the combination of itraconazole and glucocorticoids is not recommended as first-line therapy, although a brief course of glucocorticoids (<2 weeks) may be used alongside itraconazole initially. High-dose inhaled corticosteroids (ICS) and biological agents are not considered first-line therapies for acute ABPA.

Table 17.6: Guideline recommendations for treatment of ABPA[30]

Greenberger regimen[31]	An initial daily dose of prednisolone 0.5 mg/kg for 2 weeks, followed by 0.5 mg/kg every other day for 6-8 weeks, with subsequent tapering by 5–10 mg every 2 weeks until complete discontinuation at 3 months
Agarwal et al high dose regimen[32,33]	Prednisolone 0.75 mg/kg/day for 6 weeks, followed by 0.5 mg/kg/day for another 6 weeks, then transitioning to a maintenance dose of 5 mg every 6 weeks for a total duration of 6–12 months
Intermediate tapering regimens[30]	Prednisolone 0.5 mg/kg, 0.25 mg/kg, and 0.125 mg/kg daily for four weeks each, then tapered by 5 mg every two weeks till discontinuation.
Newly diagnosed ABPA[30]	Oral glucocorticoids or itraconazole (4 months)
Acute ABPA[30]	• Oral prednisolone 0.5 mg/kg/day for 2–4 weeks tapered over 4 months. • Oral itraconazole for 4 months serves as an alternative for patients where systemic glucocorticoids are contraindicated.
Exacerbations of ABPA[30]	• **First:** Oral glucocorticoids or itraconazole (4 months). • **Frequent:** Combination of oral prednisolone and itraconazole for 4 months
Treatment-dependent ABPA[30]	• Itraconazole, nebulized amphotericin B, and biologics • Low-dose glucocorticosteroids are considered the least favorable course of action in this scenario.
ABPA in remission[30]	• Management focuses on controlling underlying asthma and bronchiectasis with established therapies like inhaled corticosteroids, bronchodilators, antibiotics, and nebulized saline. • Additionally, regular monitoring with clinical reviews, serum IgE, and lung function tests (initially every 3–6 months, then every 6–12 months) is crucial. • For patients achieving remission on antifungal azoles or biologics, periodic evaluations are recommended to assess the ongoing need for these medications.

In managing subsequent flare-ups of allergic bronchopulmonary aspergillosis (ABPA), the approach mirrors that of initial treatment for newly diagnosed cases. However, for patients experiencing recurrent ABPA exacerbations (defined as two or more episodes within the past 1–2 years), a combination of oral prednisolone and the antifungal medication itraconazole becomes the recommended course of action. It is important to note that current guidelines advise against the use of biological agents and nebulized amphotericin B for treating acute ABPA exacerbations. If ABPA becomes treatment-dependent, long-term management options like itraconazole, nebulized amphotericin B, and biologics become more relevant. Importantly, continuous use of low-dose glucocorticosteroids is considered the least favorable course of action in this scenario.

PCP PNEUMONIA

For patients with proven or suspected PCP and moderate-to-severe disease (room air PaO_2 <70 mmHg or $PaO_2 - PaCO_2$ > 35 mmHg), adjunctive corticosteroids are strongly recommended to improve oxygenation and survival rates. Early initiation, ideally within 72 hours of starting PCP-specific antibiotics, is crucial for optimal benefit. The standard 21-day oral regimen for adults involves prednisone at 40 mg twice daily for the first five days, followed by a tapering schedule of 40 mg once daily for days six to ten and 20 mg once daily for days eleven to twenty-one (Table 17.7). For children with severe PCP, a similar tapering regimen is recommended, with a starting dose of 1 mg/kg twice daily for days one to five, followed by 1 mg/kg once daily for days six to ten and 0.5 mg/kg once daily for days eleven to twenty-one.[34] Intravenous methylprednisolone can be used at 75% of the prednisone dose if oral administration is not tolerated. Corticosteroids are believed to improve oxygenation by reducing inflammation in the lungs.

Table 17.7: Treatment of PCP pneumonia[34]

Age group	*Days 1–5*	*Days 6–10*	*Days 11–21*
Adults	40 mg twice daily	40 mg once daily	20 mg once daily
Children (severe PCP)	1 mg/kg twice daily	1 mg/kg once daily	0.5 mg/kg once daily

IMMUNE RECONSTITUTION INFLAMMATORY SYNDROME (IRIS)

In the context of mild immune reconstitution inflammatory syndrome (IRIS), clinicians can reassure patients experiencing minor symptoms. These symptoms actually indicate immune recovery rather than HIV progression and typically resolve with standard treatment. Treatment focuses on reducing the underlying opportunistic infection (OI) burden and managing inflammation. Nonsteroidal anti-inflammatory drugs (NSAIDs) can address discomfort from fever or minor inflammation. Drainage of abscesses, excision of inflamed lymph nodes, and inhaled steroids for cough or bronchospasm associated with mild lung inflammation may also be employed.

Severe IRIS poses a significant risk, potentially causing permanent disability or compromising a patient's functional status. Examples include vision loss from CMV retinitis, neurological complications from cryptococcal infection, or a decline in lung function due to *Mycobacterium avium* complex (MAC) or tuberculosis (TB) infection. Corticosteroid therapy is the mainstay treatment for severe IRIS, aiming to suppress the inflammatory response. While studies on corticosteroid effectiveness are limited, evidence suggests benefit in specific cases like paradoxical TB-IRIS and MAC-IRIS. Although optimal dosing regimens have not been established in trials, the guidelines committee recommends starting with prednisone (or equivalent) at 1–2 mg/kg for 1–2 weeks, followed by an individualized tapering schedule.[35,36] During the taper, if symptoms flare, the dose can be increased, and the taper can be slowed down. It is crucial to differentiate between IRIS flare and potential disease progression due to inadequate treatment of the underlying infection.

The decision to use corticosteroids must carefully weigh the potential benefits against the associated risks, particularly considering the high prevalence of type 2 diabetes, hypertension, and mental health disorders in HIV patients. Corticosteroid use can lead to hyperglycemia, hypertension, mood changes, avascular necrosis, and worsen or predispose patients to new infections. In most cases, even with IRIS, continuing antiretroviral therapy (ART) is crucial. Only in life-threatening scenarios where corticosteroids prove ineffective, particularly for central nervous system (CNS)-IRIS, might ART interruption be considered. However, this decision requires careful evaluation by an experienced HIV specialist due to the associated risks of acquiring new infections, IRIS recurrence upon ART restart, and potential development of HIV drug resistance.[35,36]

TUBERCULOSIS

Current guidelines cautiously endorse corticosteroids for specific scenarios in tuberculosis due to their anti-inflammatory effects. These include tuberculous meningitis (adjunctive therapy with dexamethasone/prednisolone to reduce mortality and disability) and pericarditis (potential benefits in reducing mortality and constrictive pericarditis risk). For tuberculous meningitis, early corticosteroid initiation demonstrably reduces mortality and disability (steroid regimens in TB, Table 17.8). While steroids are not routinely used in pulmonary TB, they can be lifesaving in severe cases like miliary TB with hypoxia or disseminated disease. However, the decision to incorporate steroids requires careful consideration of individual patient factors, balancing potential benefits against risks, and close monitoring for adverse events.

SARCOIDOSIS

The 1999 ERS/ATS/WASOG guidelines provided a robust framework for diagnosing and managing sarcoidosis.[42] Recognizing the need for ongoing advancements, the ERS assembled a dedicated Task Force in 2021. Through a meticulous review of current evidence, they formulated new guidelines encompassing not only pulmonary, cutaneous, cardiac, and neurological aspects, but also addressed sarcoidosis-associated fatigue (SAF) and small-fiber neuropathy (SFN).[43]

Glucocorticosteroids (GCs) remain the mainstay of therapy for both pulmonary and extrapulmonary sarcoidosis. While the optimal dose has not been definitively established by clinical trials, prednisone at 20–40 mg daily serves as a well-accepted starting point. This initial dose is then meticulously tapered to the lowest level that effectively controls symptoms, ideally reaching below 10 mg daily. Importantly, maintaining this lower dose regimen for an extended period of 6–24 months significantly reduces the risk of relapse associated with premature discontinuation of steroid therapy.[44]

Table 17.8: Steroid regimens for different forms of tuberculosis

Type of TB	*Steroid doses and duration*
TB meningitis[37]	**Initial:** IV dexamethasone 0.4 mg/kg/day divided into 3–4 doses (hospitalization). • *Alternatives:* Oral dexamethasone 0.4 mg/kg/day divided doses or prednisone 1 mg/kg/day single morning dose. Upon discharge, initiate a tapering regimen of oral corticosteroids for a total duration of 8–12 weeks (e.g. IV dexamethasone 0.4 mg/kg × 2 weeks → 0.3 mg/kg × 1 week → 0.2 mg/kg × 1 week → followed by 4 mg/day × 1 week → 3 mg/day × 1 week → 2 mg/day × 1 week → 1 mg/day × 1 week). (18
TB pericarditis[37]	• Prednisone was administered at 1 mg/kg daily for 4 weeks, followed by a gradual taper to 0.5 mg/kg daily for another 4 weeks before further gradual tapering over 2–4 weeks. • Alternatively, an equivalent prednisolone regimen can be employed, starting with 60 mg/day for 4 weeks, then 30 mg/day for 4 weeks, tapered to 15 mg/day for 2 weeks, followed by 5 mg/day for 1 week, and stop. • The total duration of systemic steroids is 11 weeks, depending on the regimen that may be used.
Intraocular TB[37]	• Oral prednisolone at 1 mg/kg/day is initiated, followed by a gradual taper based on individual clinical response.
Adrenal gland TB[37–40]	• Lifelong hormone replacement therapy with both glucocorticoids and mineralocorticoids becomes essential. • For mineralocorticoid replacement, once-daily fludrocortisone (0.05–0.2 mg) is commonly used. • For glucocorticoid replacement, common choices include hydrocortisone (15–25 mg in 2–3 divided doses, with the largest dose in the morning, e.g. 10 mg at waking, 5 mg mid-day, and 2.5 mg late afternoon at 6 pm to mimic the natural cortisol rhythm), prednisone (5 mg orally at bedtime), or dexamethasone (0.75 mg orally at bedtime). • Children typically receive hydrocortisone at around 8 mg/m^2/day.
TB IRIS[35,41]	• Prednisolone dosing may be employed in a stepwise manner, starting at 1.5 mg/kg orally for 2 weeks, followed by 0.75 mg/ kg orally for 2 weeks, and then gradual tapering based on individual response. • Stopping either TB therapy or ART is contraindicated.
Pediatric TB[37]	• Miliary and endobronchial TB: Recommended regimens typically involve prednisone (2 mg/kg/day) or dexamethasone (0.6 mg/kg/day) for 4 weeks, followed by a gradual 4-week taper, applicable to both miliary and endobronchial TB. • TB meningitis: For TB meningitis, prednisone (2 mg/kg/day) with a 4-week taper is advised.

HYPERSENSITIVITY PNEUMONITIS

The ATS/JRS/ALAT[45] and CHEST[46] recently published guidelines for diagnosing hypersensitivity pneumonitis (HP), which offer a standardized approach for this complex ILD. These guidelines emphasize a multidisciplinary evaluation that considers clinical symptoms, environmental exposure history, chest imaging, and potentially bronchoalveolar lavage (BAL) and lung biopsy findings, potentially leading to improved diagnostic accuracy, earlier intervention, and better patient outcomes.

A definitive treatment regimen for HP remains elusive due to limited evidence. Clinicians often employ a phenotype-based approach. For non-fibrotic HP, with the causative agent eliminated and preserved lung function, close monitoring might suffice without initial therapy. However, for patients with severe lung function decline or progressive disease, corticosteroids become a consideration. Prednisone at a dose of 40–60 mg (0.5 mg/kg/day) daily, tapering until maintenance of 10 mg/day over 2–4 weeks, offers symptom relief and improved PFTs in non-fibrotic HP.[47] Immunosuppression may be explored in fibrotic HP with severe or progressive features, although its efficacy in slowing fibrosis is not established. Corticosteroids, either alone or combined with azathioprine (AZA) or mycophenolate mofetil (MMF), remain the most frequently employed immunosuppressants in this setting. Nintedanib, a tyrosine kinase inhibitor, offers a validated treatment option for progressive fibrotic HP.

ILD

For ILDs with prominent inflammatory and autoimmune components, corticosteroids remain a cornerstone of therapy, targeting organ injury through their immunomodulatory effects. Methylprednisolone, prednisone, dexamethasone, and hydrocortisone are the most common agents, employed in both parenteral and oral forms. Two main dosing strategies exist pulse therapy with high doses for short-term control of acute exacerbations and long-term low-dose maintenance therapy for chronic disease control with minimal side effects.

IPF is the most common ILD and has a rapidly progressive course associated with deteriorating quality of life and poor prognosis. The emergence of potent antifibrotic agents like pirfenidone and nintedanib, demonstrably slowing disease progression in RCTs, has effectively relegated steroids to a backseat role in IPF treatment. Lymphocytic interstitial pneumonia and non-specific interstitial pneumonia (NSIP) have better responses to corticosteroids than usual interstitial pneumonia (UIP). The dose and duration need to be individualized (Table 17.9). Corticosteroids (CS) remain a mainstay

Table 17.9: Steroid doses for non-IPF idiopathic interstitial pneumonias (IIPs)

IIP type	*Prednisolone dose*
NSIP[51]	• 0.5–1 mg/kg/day prednisolone, not exceeding 60 mg daily, for a one-month duration. This is followed by a maintenance dose of 30–40 mg daily for an additional two months, followed by gradual tapering over 6–9 months, aiming for a final dose of 5–10 mg daily or every other day. • For acute cases with rapid respiratory failure, pulse therapy with methylprednisolone 1 g/day for 3 days, followed by 1 mg/kg/day for 4 weeks, with further tapering, is recommended.
OP[52,53]	• Prednisolone at 1–1.5 mg/kg/day, weaning over 6–12 months has demonstrated efficacy in resolving symptoms for most patients with OP. • For severe cases with respiratory failure, pulsed intravenous methylprednisolone 500–1000 mg/day for 3 days, followed by oral prednisolone 20 mg/day for 3 months with tapering attempts, and other immunosuppressive drugs (e.g. cyclophosphamide, azathioprine, cyclosporine A, mycophenolate mofetil, and rituximab), usually in combination with glucocorticoids is often employed. • Relapses are managed with either low-dose steroids or a combination of steroids and clarithromycin.

(Contd.)

Table 17.9: Steroid doses for non-IPF idiopathic interstitial pneumonias (IIPs) *(Contd.)*

IIP type	*Prednisolone dose*
LIP[54–58]	• For iLIP 1 mg/kg/day of prednisolone for 8–12 weeks, followed by tapering, with a typical treatment duration of 6–12 months. • For Sjögren's syndrome related LIP therapy with glucocorticoid and cyclophosphamide may be effective. • For HIV LIP, antiretroviral therapy (ART) serves as the first-line treatment. However, in refractory cases, corticosteroids may be cautiously considered despite potential immune suppression. • For common variable immunodeficiency (CVID) LIP corticosteroids (0.3 mg/kg equivalent prednisone) and intravenous immunoglobulin (IVIg).
DIP/RBILD[51,59]	• Smoking cessation remains the cornerstone of therapy for DIP and RBILD. • 0.5–1 mg/kg/day for 6–8 weeks, followed by tapering to 5–10 mg, are commonly employed.
AIP	• Pulse therapy (methylprednisolone 0.5–1 g/day for 3 days) followed by oral prednisolone.

in managing acute exacerbations of IPF, despite the absence of high-quality evidence from randomized controlled trials. An international survey reported widespread use of pulse methylprednisolone (500–1000 mg intravenously for 3 days) followed by oral prednisolone (1 mg/kg/day) for an average of 13 weeks.[48] This approach was mirrored in a retrospective study of 89 ILD patients (including IPF and non-IPF) with exacerbations. Optimal tapering strategies for CS in ILD exacerbations remain unclear. While gradual tapering is common, the ideal pace is debated. One study linked early tapering (10% reduction within 2 weeks) to improved outcomes in IPF exacerbations.[49,50]

CONNECTIVE TISSUE DISEASES ILD

Corticosteroids are a cornerstone therapy for ILD in connective tissue diseases (CTDs). In most CTDs except systemic sclerosis (SSc), initial treatment involves oral prednisolone starting at 0.5–1 mg/kg. The aim is to gradually taper this dose to a low maintenance level of 10 mg/day or less. This approach is often combined with immunosuppressant medication, such as cyclophosphamide (oral or intravenous) or azathioprine, for enhanced disease control.

Corticosteroids are a mainstay in managing both rheumatoid arthritis (RA) and SLE manifestations. For RA-ILD, prednisone is the preferred glucocorticosteroid, typically starting at 0.5 mg/kg/day for 6–8 weeks before tapering and transitioning to DMARDs for long-term disease control (Table 17.10). Methylprednisolone may be used in pulse therapy for rapidly progressive RA.[60] In SLE, initial treatment involves prednisolone or methylprednisolone at doses ranging from 0.5 to 1 mg/kg/day orally or 0.5 to 1 gm intravenously daily for 3 days in pulse therapy. The goal is to taper prednisolone to a minimal dose of 7.5–5 mg/day while introducing steroid-sparing medications like MMF, azathioprine, belimumab, rituximab, or tacrolimus for long-term control.[61] ILD associated with polymyositis/dermatomyositis may necessitate earlier intervention. Here, higher prednisolone doses (0.75–1 mg/kg) alongside cyclophosphamide or another immunosuppressant are used to prevent disease progression.[62] Conversely,

Table 17.10: Proposed therapies for CTD-ILD[66]		
Medication	*Dose*	*Disease*
SoluMedrol	500–1000 mg/day IV × 3 days	Acute ILD in RA, IIMs, SS
Prednisone	1 mg/kg/day up to 60 mg	Subacute ILD in RA, IIMs, SS
Mycophenolate mofetil	2000–3000 mg/day divided doses	RA, SSc, IIMs, SS
Mycophenolic acid	720–1080 mg b.d.	ILD in SS
Azathioprine	2–3 mg/kg/day	RA, SSc, IIMs
Tacrolimus	1–3 mg/day	ILD in IIMs
Cyclophosphamide	**IV monthly:** 750 mg/m^2 × 6 months **Oral:** 1.5–2.5 mg/kg/day	RA, SSc, IIMs
Rituximab	1000 mg IV × 2, then q6 months	RA, SSc, IIMs
Nintedanib	150 mg PO twice daily	RA, SSc, IIMs

SSc-ILD requires a more cautious approach. Treatment, if needed, typically involves lower prednisolone doses (around 10 mg/day) with the possible addition of cyclophosphamide.[63–65] High-dose prednisolone (exceeding 10 mg/day) is strongly discouraged due to the increased risk of renal crisis.

ANCA-ASSOCIATED VASCULITIS (AAV)

The 2016 EULAR recommendations for ANCA-associated vasculitis (AAV) management combined treatment approaches for granulomatosis with polyangiitis (GPA) and microscopic polyangiitis (MPA) with eosinophilic granulomatosis with polyangiitis (EGPA). This reflected a stronger evidence base for GPA/MPA therapies. However, recent randomized controlled trials (RCTs) support more specific treatment strategies for EGPA, necessitating separate treatment recommendations for this condition. Furthermore, advancements in ANCA testing warrant updated diagnostic procedure recommendations. An international effort by the European Vasculitis Society recently led to a revised international consensus for ANCA testing, prompting the need to revisit the 2016 EULAR guidelines on AAV diagnostics.[67]

Building on these developments, the 2022 EULAR recommendations incorporate recent evidence through three systematic literature reviews (SLRs) covering: AAV treatment (including EGPA), diagnostic testing and follow-up procedures for AAV, general AAV management.[68]

Treatment of GPA/MPA

Remission induction in non-severe GPA and MPA: Treatment with a combination of GC and RTX is recommended for induction of remission of non-organ- or non-life-threatening GPA/MPA. For remission, induction in GPA/MPA, oral GC treatment starts from a dose of 50–75 mg prednisolone/day. A stepwise dose reduction is recommended to achieve 5 mg prednisolone/day dosage by 4–5 months (Table 17.11). In GPA/MPA, RTX maintenance is recommended after remission induction with either RTX or CYC. PLEX (plasma exchange) may be considered for remission induction in GPA/MPA for patients with serum creatinine >300 µmol/L and active glomerulonephritis. Routine

Table 17.11: Treatment of GPA/MPA[68]	
Remission induction for non-severe GPA/MPA[69]	Oral GC treatment starts from a dose of 50–75 mg prednisolone/day. A stepwise dose reduction is recommended to achieve 5 mg prednisolone/day dosage by 4–5 months.
Life-threatening GPA/MPA[70]	Pulsed methylprednisolone therapy (1000–3000 mg daily for 3–5 days) followed by oral glucocorticoids 1 mg/kg daily prednisone (or equivalent) and rapid dose reduction to 20 mg daily by 7 weeks and 5 mg daily by 19 weeks is equally effective and safer than traditional high-dose regimens (the PEXIVAS trial).
For relapsing cases[71,72]	Glucocorticoids with rituximab (The RITAZAREM trial) glucocorticoids at lower initial doses, such as 0.5 mg/kg daily, even for severe disease, with maintenance rituximab at 1,000 mg every 4 months over 2 years[73,74]
Maintenance of remission[73]	Rituximab or cyclophosphamide for 24–48 months following induction, along with low-dose steroids. According to the MAINRITSAN trail, the recommended dosage of rituximab for remission maintenance is 500 mg every 6 months for 18 to 36 months.

use is not recommended to treat alveolar hemorrhage in GPA/MPA. Avacopan: For patients requiring reduced GC exposure, avacopan may be considered in combination with RTX or CYC for remission induction in GPA/MPA.

EGPA

Early diagnosis and treatment are crucial in EGPA, as untreated patients have a high mortality rate. The choice of therapy depends on disease severity. For patients with mild disease, corticosteroids like prednisone (1–1.5 mg/kg/day or 60 mg/day in adults) are the mainstay of treatment, aiming to control symptoms and achieve remission. The dose is then tapered slowly (e.g. 5–10 mg daily) for up to a year to minimize side effects (Table 17.12). Patients with severe disease features like cardiac or renal involvement often receive high-dose corticosteroids like methylprednisolone (15 mg/kg/day) may be needed initially, often combined with immunosuppressants like cyclophosphamide to improve survival. Cyclophosphamide use requires close monitoring for potential side effects. Azathioprine (2 mg/kg/day) can be used for maintenance therapy after remission is achieved in recent years, drugs targeting the IL-5 pathway, such as mepolizumab (300 mg every 4 weeks), have emerged as effective treatment options with fewer side effects compared to traditional corticosteroids. Other treatment modalities like intravenous immunoglobulin (IVIg) and interferon-α (IFN-α) may be considered in specific situations like pregnancy or severe organ involvement, but their use is limited due to variable efficacy and potential side effects. Prophylaxis for *Pneumocystis jirovecii* pneumonia is recommended for patients on prolonged high-dose corticosteroids and other immunosuppressants.

2022 EULAR Recommendations for EGPA[68]

- High-dose GC and CYC combination recommended for remission induction of new-onset or relapsing EGPA with organ- or life-threatening manifestations.
- GC recommended for remission induction in new-onset or relapsing EGPA without organ- or life-threatening manifestations.
- **MEP (mepolizumab):** Recommended in patients with relapsing or refractory EGPA without active organ- or life-threatening disease. Recommended at the time of relapse

Table 17.12: EGPA treatment regimens[68]	
Remission induction non-life-threatening manifestations[74–76]	
FFS = 0	Prednisolone at 1 mg/kg/day for 3 weeks (maximum 80 mg/day), followed by a gradual tapering schedule: 7.5 mg reduction every two weeks until reaching 0.25 mg/kg/day after 3 months, then 5 mg reduction every 2 weeks until 10 mg/day, and finally 1 mg reduction every 3 weeks to the lowest effective dose.
FFS ≥1	Rituximab (1000 mg pulses every 2 weeks) + low-dose prednisone (≤7.5 mg daily) or cyclophosphamide (nine pulses over five months) + low-dose prednisone (≤7.5 mg daily)
FFS >2	Additional immunosuppressive therapy with cyclophosphamide to improve survival.
Life-threatening manifestations[77,78]	
Remission induction	High-dose corticosteroids + cyclophosphamide (600 mg/m^2 on days 1, 15, 29; then 500 mg every 15–20 days) or rituximab (1 g on days 1 and 15)
Remission maintenance	Methotrexate (15–20 mg weekly), azathioprine (2 mg/kg/day), mepolizumab, rituximab
Relapse/refractory manifestations[79]	
Respiratory (initial)	Topical bronchodilators + low-dose oral steroids
Respiratory (unresponsive)	Short course of high-dose steroids (0.5–1 mg/kg/day for 5–7 days) + mepolizumab (if needed)
ENT (relapsing)	Functional endoscopic sinus surgery (FESS)
Systemic	Mepolizumab (300 mg every 4 weeks) + low-dose steroids
Maintenance of remission of relapsing EGPA of non-life-threatening and life-threatening manifestations—glucocorticoids and mepolizumab.	
Special conditions like pregnancy—glucocorticoids, intravenous immunoglobulins (IVIg), and interferon-α (IFN-α) and azathioprine are relatively safe.	

for maintenance remission of relapsing EGPA after induction remission for non-organ- or life-threatening manifestations.

- **Assays for ANCA testing :** Testing for both PR3-and MPO-ANCA using high-quality antigen-specific assay as a primary test recommended.
- ***Pneumocystis jirovecii* prophylaxis:** Recommend the use of TMP/SMX as prophylaxis against *Pneumocystis jirovecii* pneumonia in patients with AAV receiving RTX, CYC and/or high doses of GC.

EOSINOPHILIC LUNG DISEASES

AEP/CEP

Corticosteroids are the mainstay treatment for both acute eosinophilic pneumonia (AEP) and chronic eosinophilic pneumonia (CEP). In AEP, the goal is to identify and eliminate the causative agent if possible. Corticosteroids induce eosinophil apoptosis and lead to disease resolution in most patients. Initial treatment typically involves intravenous methylprednisolone at doses ranging from 60 to 125 mg administered every 6 hours. After respiratory failure resolves, patients are transitioned to oral prednisone (40–60 mg/day) for 2–4 weeks with a gradual taper over several weeks.[79] Unlike AEP, CEP requires long-term corticosteroid therapy for disease control. A recommended regimen starts with prednisone 0.5 mg/kg/day (40–60 mg daily) continued for 4–6 weeks until symptoms and radiographic abnormalities resolve. The dose is then slowly tapered, followed by maintenance for at least 3 months, ideally up to 9 months, with gradual reductions every 4 weeks.[80] Shorter prednisone courses may also be effective. Despite the effectiveness of corticosteroids, relapses are common in CEP, potentially requiring increased prednisone doses (up to 40 mg/day) for relapse management. Inhaled steroids are not effective for CEP but may be used to prevent relapses in patients with asthma. Newer biologic agents targeting the IL-5 pathway, like mepolizumab, are emerging as steroid-sparing options for CEP.

Hypereosinophilic Syndrome (HES)

Prior to effective therapies, hypereosinophilic syndrome (HES) had a poor prognosis, with most patients succumbing within a year of diagnosis. Fortunately, treatment advancements have significantly improved median survival to over 10 years. The course of HES and treatment options depend on the underlying cause and severity. In life-threatening cases with high eosinophil counts (over 100,000/μl) or cardiac/neurologic involvement, prompt initiation of corticosteroids (prednisone 1 mg/kg/day to methylprednisolone 1 g) is crucial while awaiting definitive diagnosis. For patients with FIP1L1-PDGFRA fusion, imatinib (initial dose 400 mg/day) is the mainstay of treatment.[81] Additionally, those with cardiac involvement should receive concurrent corticosteroids to prevent further damage. In cases of resistance to imatinib, alternative tyrosine kinase inhibitors like nilotinib or sorafenib can be explored. For patients lacking FIP1L1-PDGFRA mutations or other targetable mutations with organ involvement, corticosteroids (prednisone 1 mg/kg/day for several weeks) are the mainstay (Table 17.13). If successful in controlling symptoms and eosinophilia, corticosteroids can be gradually tapered to an alternate-day schedule and continued for about a year at the lowest effective dose. Mepolizumab (300 mg every 4 weeks), an anti-IL-5 antibody, has shown promise in reducing flares for patients with HES negative for FIP1L1-PDGFRA. Other treatment options include interferon-α (as a second-line agent or steroid-sparing

Table 17.13: Management of hypereosinophilic syndromes (HES)

HES variant	*Initial therapy*	*Maintenance therapy*	*Duration*
FIP1L1-PDGFRA fusion positive[81]	Imatinib mesylate 100 mg per day + Prednisolone 1 mg/kg/day (first few days only)	Imatinib mesylate maintenance dose	Until sustained remission
FIP1L1-PDGFRA fusion negative (no imatinib response)[82] Lymphoid HES Idiopathic HES	Prednisolone 1 mg/kg/day	Prednisolone tapered to every-other-day schedule	Approximately 1 year
Corticosteroid-resistant or severe cases	Individualized based on response and tolerability	Hydroxyurea, interferon-α, cyclosporine A, alemtuzumab	As needed

therapy) and hydroxyurea (0.5–1.5 g/day) added to the regimen for steroid-refractory disease or toxicity. Vincristine may be used in severe cases with extremely high white blood cell counts. Newer agents like JAK inhibitors (tofacitinib, ruxolitinib) and anti-CD52 antibody alemtuzumab are showing some success in specific variants of HES but require further investigation. Allogeneic bone marrow transplantation is reserved for severe cases with potentially reversible organ damage.

Radiation Pneumonitis

Systemic corticosteroids, typically prednisolone at 0.5–1 mg/kg/day for 2 weeks followed by a gradual taper, currently serve as the cornerstone of therapy for acute radiation pneumonitis.[83]

LUNG TRANSPLANTATION

In lung transplantation, corticosteroids play a crucial role as part of the immunosuppressive regimen. Immediately upon successful reperfusion of the donor allograft (i.e. connection of its blood vessels and bronchus to the recipient), a high-dose intravenous bolus of methylprednisolone (500–1000 mg) is administered (Table 17.14). Maintenance therapy then commences with oral prednisone (or equivalent) at a dose of 0.5–1 mg/kg/day, followed by gradual tapering within 6 months to reach a target maintenance dose of 5–10 mg/day. This tapering aims to balance the immunosuppressive effect with minimizing long-term steroid-related complications. Corticosteroids, along with azathioprine, remain one of the oldest-used immunosuppressants in any solid organ transplant.[84] Intravenous methylprednisolone and oral prednisone are the most used corticosteroids for the prevention and treatment of rejection.

Table 17.14: Corticosteroids in lung transplantation

Stage	*Corticosteroid*	*Dose*	*Duration*
Induction (upon reperfusion)	Methylprednisolone	500–1000 mg bolus	Immediately after reperfusion
Maintenance	Prednisone (or equivalent)	0.5–1 mg/kg/day	6 months with gradual tapering to reach a target maintenance dose of 5–10 mg/day

REFERENCES

1. Melani AS, Croce S, Cassai L. et al. Systemic Corticosteroids for Treating Respiratory Diseases: Less is Better, but… When and How is it Possible in Real Life?. Pulm Ther 2023;9:329–344. https://doi.org/10.1007/s41030-023-00227-x.
2. Metlay JP, Waterer GW, Long AC, et al. Diagnosis and treatment of adults with community-acquired pneumonia an Official Clinical Practice Guideline of the American Thoracic Society and Infectious Diseases Society of America. *Am J Respir Crit Care Med.* 2019;200(7):e45–67. https://doi.org/10.1164/rccm.201908-1581ST. (PMID: 31573350).
3. Menéndez R, Torres A, Asp J, et al. Community-acquired Pneumonia. New Guidelines of the Spanish Society of Pulmonology and Thoracic Surgery (SEPAR) Neumología adquirida en la comunidad. Nueva normativa de la Sociedad Española de Neumología y Cirugía Torácica (SEPAR). Arch Bronconeumol. 2010;46(10):543–58.
4. Boyles TH, Brink A, Calligaro GL, et al. South African guideline for the management of community-acquired pneumonia in adults. *J Thorac Dis.* 2017;9:1469–502.

5. Martin-Loeches I, Torres A, Nagavci B, et al. ERS/ESICM/ESCMID/ALAT guidelines for the management of severe community-acquired pneumonia. *Eur Respir J*. 2023;61(4):2200735. https://doi.org/10.1183/13993003.00735-2022. (PMID: 37012080).
6. EMA. https://www.ema.europa.eu/en/news/ema-endorses-use-dexamethasone-covid-19-patients-oxygen-mechanical-ventilation. Accessed 15 Jan 2023.
7. World Health Organization. Corticosteroids for COVID-19: Living guidance 2 September 2020. https://www.who.int/publications-detail-redirect/WHO-2019-nCoV-Corticosteroids-2020.1. Accessed 15 Jan 2023.
8. IDSA. https://www.idsociety.org/practice-guideline/covid-19-guideline-treatment-and-management/#null COVID-19 Treatment Guidelines Panel. Coronavirus Disease 2019 (COVID-19) Treatment Guidelines. Accessed 15 Jan 2023.
9. Roche N, Crichton ML, Goeminne PC, et al. Update June 2022: management of hospitalised adults with coronavirus disease 2019 (COVID-19): a European Respiratory Society living guideline. *Eur Respir J*. 2022;60(2):2200803. https://doi.org/10.1183/13993003.00803-2022. (PMID: 35710264).
10. National Institutes of Health. COVID-19 Treatment Guidelines Panel. Coronavirus Disease 2019 (COVID-19) Treatment Guidelines. National Institutes of Health. https://www.COVID-19treatmentguidelines.nih.gov/. Accessed 15 Jan 2023.
11. Global Initiative for Asthma. Global strategy for asthma management and prevention. Available from https://ginasthma.org/wp-content/uploads/2021/04/GINA-2021-MainReport_FINAL_21_04_28-WMS.pdf. Accessed 24 Jan 2023.
12. Ramsahai JM, Hansbro PM, Wark PAB. Mechanisms and management of asthma exacerbations. Am *J Respir Crit Care Med*. 2019;199(4):423–32. https://doi.org/10.1164/rccm.201810-1931CI. (PMID: 30562041).
13. Paton J, White J, Annandale J, et al. British guideline on the management of asthma. London: British Thoracic Society and Scottish Intercollegiate Guideline Network; 2019.
14. Rothe T, Spagnolo P, Bridevaux PO, et al. Diagnosis and management of asthma—the Swiss Guidelines. Respiration. 2018;95(5):364–80. https://doi.org/10.1159/000486797. (PMID: 29614508).
15. NHLBI Asthma Management Guidelines: Focused Updates 2020. https://www.nhlbi.nih.gov/health-topics/asthma-management-guidelines-2020-updates. Accessed 23 Jan 2023.
16. Nan C, Schmidt O, Lindner R, et al. German regional variation of acute and high oral corticosteroid use for asthma. J Asthma. 2022;59(4):791–800. https://doi.org/10.1080/02770903.2021.1878532. (PMID: 33492176).
17. Blakey J, Chung LP, McDonald VM, et al. Oral corticosteroids stewardship for asthma in adults and adolescents: A position paper from the Thoracic Society of Australia and New Zealand. Respirology. 2021;26(12):1112–30. https://doi.org/10.1111/resp.14147. (PMID: 34587348).
18. Global Initiative for Chronic Obstructive Lung Disease. Global strategy for the diagnosis, management, and prevention of chronic obstructive lung disease. Updated 2023. http://www.goldcopd.org/uploads/users/files/GOLD_Report.pdf. Accessed 12 Jan 2023.
19. Wedzicha JA, Miravitlles M, Hurst JR, et al. Management of COPD exacerbations: an ERS/ATS guideline. *Eur Respir J*. 2017;49:1600791.
20. NICE. Chronic obstructive pulmonary disease in over 16s: diagnosis and management. Evidence reviews for the length of corticosteroid use during exacerbations NICE guideline NG115 2019. https://www.nice.org.uk/guidance/ng115/evidence/j-length-of-corticosteroid-use-during-exacerbations-pdf-237699674965. Accessed 12 Jan 2023.
21. Canadian Respiratory Guidelines. COPD action plan. https://cts-sct.ca/wp-content/uploads/2019/03/5491_THOR_COPDActionPlanUpdate_2019_Editable_Eng_v2.pdf. Accessed 12 Jan 2023.
22. Japanese Respiratory Society. Guidelines for the Diagnosis and Treatment of COPD. 3rd edition. 2010. http://www.jrs.or.jp/uploads/uploads/files/photos/765.pdf 61. Accessed 12 Jan 2023.
23. Thoracic Society of Australia and New Zealand. The COPD-X plan. http://copdx.org.au/copd-x-plan/. Accessed 12 Jan 2023.

24. Miravitlles M, Calle M, Molina J, for the Spanish Guideline for COPD (GesEPOC), et al. Spanish COPD guidelines (GesEPOC) 2021: updated pharmacological treatment of stable COPD. Arch Bronconeumol. 2022;58: T69–81.
25. Griffiths MJ, McAuley DF, Perkins GD, et al. Guidelines on the management of acute respiratory distress syndrome. BMJ Open Respir Res. 2019;6: e000420.
26. Papazian L, Aubron C, Brochard L, et al. Formal guidelines: management of acute respiratory distress syndrome. Ann Intensive Care. 2019;9(1):69. https://doi.org/10.1186/s13613-019-0540-9. (PMID: 31197492).
27. Tasaka S, Ohshimo S, Takeuchi M, on behalf of the ARDS Clinical Practice Guideline 2021 committee from the Japanese Society of Intensive Care Medicine, the Japanese Respiratory Society, and the Japanese Society of Respiratory Care Medicine, et al. ARDS clinical practice guideline 2021. *J Intensive Care*. 2022;10(1):32. https://doi.org/10.1186/s40560-022-00615-6. (PMID: 35799288).
28. Liang H, Song H, Zhai R, et al. Corticosteroids for treating sepsis in adult patients: a systematic review and meta-analysis. Front Immunol. 2021; 12:709155. https://doi.org/10.3389/fimmu.2021.709155. (PMID: 34484209).
29. Agarwal R, Chakrabarti A, Shah A, Gupta D, Meis JF, Guleria R, Moss R, Denning DW; ABPA complicating asthma ISHAM working group. Allergic bronchopulmonary aspergillosis: review of literature and proposal of new diagnostic and classification criteria. Clin Exp Allergy. 2013 Aug;43(8):850–73. doi: 10.1111/cea.12141. PMID: 23889240.
30. Agarwal R, Sehgal IS, Muthu V, Denning DW, Chakrabarti A, Soundappan K, ..., Aggarwal AN. (2024). Revised clinical practice guidelines for diagnosing, classifying, and treating allergic bronchopulmonary aspergillosis/mycoses: a Delphi statement from the ISHAM-ABPA working group. *European Respiratory Journal*.
31. Greenberger PA. Allergic bronchopulmonary aspergillosis. J Allergy Clin Immunol. 2002;110:685–692.
32. Agarwal R. Allergic bronchopulmonary aspergillosis. Chest. 2009;135:805–826.
33. Agarwal R, Gupta D, Agarwal AN, et al. Allergic bronchopulmonary aspergillosis: lessons from 126 patients attending chest clinic in north India. Chest. 2006; 130:442–448.
34. Quigley N, d'Amours L, Gervais P, Dion G. (2024, January). Epidemiology, Risk Factors, and Prophylaxis Use for Pneumocystis jirovecii Pneumonia in the Non-HIV Population: A Retrospective Study in Québec, Canada. In Open Forum Infectious Diseases (Vol. 11, No. 1, p. ofad639). US: Oxford University Press.
35. Brust JCM, McGowan JP, Fine SM, et al. Management of IRIS [Internet]. Baltimore (MD): Johns Hopkins University; 2024 Mar.
36. Yadav S, Rawal G, Jeyaraman M (2023). Tuberculosis of the navicular bone of the left foot without pulmonary involvement in a fifteen-year-old indian boy: a rare case report. Cureus, 15(6).
37. Gupta S, Ansari MAM, Gupta AK, Chaudhary P, Bansal LK. Current Approach for Diagnosis and Treatment of Adrenal Tuberculosis-Our Experience and Review of Literature. Surg J (N Y). 2022 Mar 3;8(1): e92–97. doi: 10.1055/s-0042-1743523. PMID: 35252566; PMCID: PMC8894089.
38. 26. Bornstein SR, Allolio B, Arlt W. Diagnosis and treatment of primary adrenal insufficiency: an Endocrine Society Clinical Practice Guideline. *J Clin Endocrinol Metab*. 2016;101(02):364–389.
39. 27. Huecker MR, Bhutta BS, Dominique E. Adrenal Insufficiency. [Updated 2023 Aug 17]. In: StatPearls [Internet]. Treasure Island (FL): StatPearls Publishing; 2024 January.
40. Quinn CM, Poplin V, Kasibante J, Yuquimpo K, Gakuru J, Cresswell FV, Bahr NC. Tuberculosis IRIS: Pathogenesis, Presentation, and Management across the Spectrum of Disease. Life (Basel). 2020 Oct 29;10(11):262. doi: 10.3390/life10110262. PMID: 33138069; PMCID: PMC7693460.
41. American Thoracic Society, European Respiratory Society (ERS), and World Association of Sarcoidosis and Other Granulomatous Disorders. Statement on sarcoidosis. Joint Statement of the American Thoracic Society (ATS), the European Respiratory Society (ERS), and the World Association of Sarcoidosis and Other Granulomatous Disorders (WASOG) adopted by the ATS Board of Directors and by the ERS Executive Committee, February 1999. *Am J Respir Crit Care Med* 1999;160:736–755. doi: 10.1164/ajrccm.160.2.ats4-99.

42. Baughman RP, Valeyre D, Korsten P, et al. ERS clinical practice guidelines on treatment of sarcoidosis. *Eur Respir J* 2021;58:2004079.
43. Rahaghi FF, Baughman RP, Saketkoo LA, et al. Delphi consensus recommendations for a treatment algorithm in pulmonary sarcoidosis. Eur Respir Rev 2020;29:190146.
44. Raghu G, Remy-Jardin M, Ryerson CJ, et al. Diagnosis of hypersensitivity pneumonitis in adults. An official ATS/JRS/ALAT clinical practice guideline. *Am J Respir Crit Care Med* 2020;202:e36–69. doi:10.1164/rccm.202005-2032ST.
45. Fernández Pérez ER, Travis WD, Lynch DA, et al. Executive summary diagnosis and evaluation of hypersensitivity pneumonitis: CHEST guideline and expert panel report. Chest 2021;160:595–615. doi:10.1016/j.chest.2021.03.067.
46. Diagnosis, course and management of hypersensitivity pneumonitis Mark Hamblin, Helmut Prosch, Martina Vašáková European Respiratory Review Mar 2022;31(163):210169; DOI: 10.1183/16000617.0169-2021.
47. Adams CJ, Chohan K, Rozenberg D, et al. Feasibility and outcomes of a standardized management protocol for acute exacerbation of interstitial lung disease. Lung. 2021;199(4):379–87. https://doi.org/10.1007/s00408-021-00463-5.
48. Anan K, Kataoka Y, Ichikado K, et al. Early corticosteroid dose tapering in patients with acute exacerbation of idiopathic pulmonary fibrosis. Respir Res. 2022;23(1):291. https://doi.org/10.1186/s12931-022-02195-3.
49. Yamazaki R, Nishiyama O, Saeki S, et al. An initial therapeutic dose of corticosteroid for an acute exacerbation of IPF is associated with subsequent early recurrence of another exacerbation. Sci Rep.2021;11:5782.
50. Nayfeh AS, Chippa V, Moore DR. Nonspecific Interstitial Pneumonia. [Updated 2023 Aug 14]. In: StatPearls [Internet]. Treasure Island (FL): StatPearls Publishing; 2024 Jan-. Available from: https://www.ncbi.nlm.nih.gov/books/NBK518974.
51. Bradley B, Branley HM, Egan JJ, Greaves MS, Hansell DM, Harrison NK, Hirani N, Hubbard R, Lake F, Millar AB, Wallace WA. Interstitial lung disease guideline: the British Thoracic Society in collaboration with the Thoracic Society of Australia and New Zealand and the Irish Thoracic Society (vol 63, Suppl V, pg v1, 2008). Thorax. 2008 Nov 1;63(11):1029-.
52. Radzikowska E, Fijolek J. Update on cryptogenic organizing pneumonia. Frontiers in Medicine. 2023 Apr 20; 10:1146782.
53. Dong X, Gao YL, Lu Y, Zheng Y. Characteristics of primary Sjögren's syndrome related lymphocytic interstitial pneumonia. Clin Rheumatol. 2021 Feb;40(2):601-612. doi: 10.1007/s10067-020-05236-8. Epub 2020 Jul 1. PMID: 32613392; PMCID: PMC7327216.
54. Tasdemir MN, Aslan S. Lymphocytic Interstitial Pneumonia in a Man with Human Immunodeficiency Virus Infection. Revista da Sociedade Brasileira de Medicina Tropical. 2023 Jun 2;56:e0055–2023.
55. Panchabhai TS, Farver C, Highland KB. Lymphocytic interstitial pneumonia. Clinics in Chest Medicine. 2016 Sep 1;37(3):463–74.
56. Hurst JR, Verma N, Lowe D, Baxendale HE, Jolles S, Kelleher P, Longhurst HJ, Patel SY, Renzoni EA, Sander CR and Avery GR. British Lung Foundation/United Kingdom Primary Immunodeficiency Network consensus statement on the definition, diagnosis, and management of granulomatous-lymphocytic interstitial lung disease in common variable immunodeficiency disorders. The Journal of Allergy and Clinical Immunology: In Practice, 2017;5(4):938–945.
57. Lamers OA, Smits BM, Leavis HL, de Bree GJ, Cunningham-Rundles C, Dalm VA, Ho HE, Hurst JR, IJspeert H, Prevaes SM, Robinson A. Treatment strategies for GLILD in common variable immunodeficiency: a systematic review. Frontiers in Immunology. 2021 Apr 15;12:606099.
58. Ryu JH, Myers JL, Capizzi SA, Douglas WW, Vassallo R, Decker PA. Desquamative interstitial pneumonia and respiratory bronchiolitis-associated interstitial lung disease. Chest. 2005 Jan 1;127(1):178–84.
59. Wells AU, Hirani N, on behalf of the British Thoracic Society Interstitial Lung Disease Guideline Group, a subgroup of the British Thoracic Society Standards of Care Committee, in collaboration with the Thoracic Society of Australia and New Zealand and the Irish Thoracic Society. Interstitial

lung disease guideline: the British Thoracic Society in collaboration with the Thoracic Society of Australia and New Zealand and the Irish Thoracic Society. Thorax. (2008) 63(Suppl V):v1–58. doi: 10.1136/thx.2008.101691.

60. Fanouriakis A, Kostopoulou M, Alunno A, Aringer M, Bajema I, Boletis JN, Cervera R, Doria A, Gordon C, Govoni M, et al. 2019 Update of the EULAR Recommendations for the Management of Systemic Lupus Erythematosus. Ann. Rheum. Dis. 2019;78:736–745. doi: 10.1136/annrheumdis-2019-215089.
61. Lundberg IE, Tjärnlund A, Bottai M, Werth VP, Pilkington C, Visser M, Alfredsson L, Amato AA, Barohn RJ, Liang MH, et al. European League Against Rheumatism/American College of Rheumatology classification criteria for adult and juvenile idiopathic inflammatory myopathies and their major subgroups. Ann. Rheum. Dis. 2017;76:1955–64.
62. Tashkin DP, Elashoff R, Clements PJ, et al. Cyclophosphamide versus placebo in scleroderma lung disease. *N Engl J Med*. 2006;354:2655–2666.
63. Tashkin DP, Roth MD, Clements PJ, et al. Mycophenolate mofetil versus oral cyclophosphamide in scleroderma-related interstitial lung disease (SLS II): a randomised controlled, double-blind, parallel-group trial. Lancet Respir Med. 2016;4:708–719.
64. Ando K, Motojima S, Doi T, et al. Effect of glucocorticoid monotherapy on pulmonary function and survival in Japanese patients with scleroderma-related interstitial lung disease. Respir Invest 2013; 51:69–75.
65. ATS Connective Tissue-related Interstitial Lung Disease Primer 2020 https://www.thoracic.org/education-center/ild/pdf/2020_ats_ctd-ild_v13_web.pdf.
66. Richette P, Doherty M, Pascual E, Barskova V, Becce F, Castañeda-Sanabria J, Coyfish M, Guillo S, Jansen TL, Janssens H, Lioté F, Mallen C, Nuki G, Perez-Ruiz F, Pimentao J, Punzi L, Pywell T, So A, Tausche AK, Uhlig T, Zavada J, Zhang W, Tubach F, Bardin T. 2016 updated EULAR evidence-based recommendations for the management of gout. Ann Rheum Dis. 2017 Jan;76(1):29-42. doi: 10.1136/annrheumdis-2016-209707. Epub 2016 Jul 25. PMID: 27457514.
67. Hellmich B, Sanchez-Alamo B, Schirmer JH, Berti A, Blockmans D, Cid MC, Holle JU, Hollinger N, Karadag O, Kronbichler A, Little MA, Luqmani RA, Mahr A, Merkel PA, Mohammad AJ, Monti S, Mukhtyar CB, Musial J, Price-Kuehne F, Segelmark M, Teng YKO, Terrier B, Tomasson G, Vaglio A, Vassilopoulos D, Verhoeven P, Jayne D. EULAR recommendations for the management of ANCA-associated vasculitis: 2022 update. Ann Rheum Dis. 2024 Jan 2;83(1):30-47. doi: 10.1136/ard-2022-223764. PMID: 36927642.
68. Antonelou M, Abro A, Heath R, et al. Comparison of outcomes using the rituximab originator MabThera with the biosimilar truxima in patients with ANCA-associated vasculitis. Scand J Rheumatol 2022;51:135–41.
69. Walsh M, et al. Plasma exchange and glucocorticoids in severe ANCA-associated vasculitis. *N. Engl. J. Med*. 2020;382:622–631. A clinical trial of induction therapies in severe AAV, demonstrates that lower-dose glucocorticoids are non-inferior to standard doses and that routine use of plasma exchange as an adjuvant provides no additional benefit.
70. Smith R, Jayne D, Merkel P. A randomized, controlled trial of rituximab versus azathioprine after induction of remission with rituximab for patients with ANCA-associated vasculitis and relapsing disease (abstract). Arthritis Rheumatol. 2019;71 (Suppl. 10).
71. Gopaluni S, et al. Rituximab versus azathioprine as therapy for maintenance of remission for antineutrophil cytoplasm antibody-associated vasculitis (RITAZAREM): study protocol for a randomized controlled trial. Trials 2017;18:112.
72. Guillevin L, Pagnoux C, Karras A, et al. Rituximab versus azathioprine for maintenance in ANCA-associated vasculitis. *N Engl J Med* 2014;371:1771–80.
73. Puechal X, Pagnoux C, Baron G, et al. Adding azathioprine to remission-induction glucocorticoids for eosinophilic granulomatosis with polyangiitis (Churg-Strauss), microscopic polyangiitis, or polyarteritis nodosa without poor prognosis factors: A randomized, controlled trial. Arthritis Rheumatol 2017;69:2175–86.

74. Ribi C, et al. Treatment of Churg-Strauss syndrome without poor prognosis factors: a multicenter, prospective, randomized, open-label study of seventy-two patients. Arthritis Rheum. 2008;58:586–594.
75. Terrier B, Pugnet G deC, et al. Rituximab versus conventional therapeutic strategy for remission induction in eosinophilic granulomatosis with polyangiitis: A double-blind, randomized, controlled trial [abstract]. Arthritis and Rheumatology 2021;73.
76. Cohen P, et al. Churg-Strauss syndrome with poor prognosis factors: a prospective multicenter trial comparing glucocorticoids and six or twelve cyclophosphamide pulses in forty-eight patients. Arthritis Care Res. 2007;57:686–693.
77. Puéchal X, et al. Non-severe eosinophilic granulomatosis with polyangiitis: long-term outcomes after remission-induction trial. Rheumatology 2019;58:2107–2116.
78. Allen JN, Pacht ER, Gadek JE, et al. Acute eosinophilic pneumonia is a reversible cause of noninfectious respiratory failure. *N Engl J Med* 1989;321:569–574.
79. Marchand E, Reynaud-Gaubert M, Lauque D, Durieu J, Tonnel AB, Cordier JF. Idiopathic chronic eosinophilic pneumonia. A clinical and follow-up study of 62 cases. The Groupe d'Etudes et de Recherche sur les Maladies "Orphelines" Pulmonaires (GERM"O"P) Medicine (Baltimore) 1998;77:299–312.
80. Cools J, DeAngelo DJ, Gotlib J, et al. A tyrosine kinase created by a fusion of the PDGFRA and FIP1L1 genes as a therapeutic target of imatinib in idiopathic hypereosinophilic syndrome. *N Engl J Med* 2003;348:1201–1214.
81. Chusid MJ, Dale DC, West BC, Wolff SM. The hypereosinophilic syndrome: analysis of fourteen cases with review of the literature. Medicine (Baltimore) 1975;54:1–27.
82. Jain V, Berman AT. Radiation pneumonitis: old problem, new tricks. Cancers (Basel). 2018;10(7):1.
83. Nelson J, Alvey N, Bowman L, Schulte J, Segovia MC, McDermott J, et al. Consensus recommendations for use of maintenance immunosuppression in solid organ transplantation: Endorsed by the American College of Clinical Pharmacy, American Society of Transplantation, and the International Society for Heart and Lung Transplantation. Pharmacotherapy. 2022 Aug 1;42(8):599–633.

Index